To Console the North Wind

Hand of the Wind Taijiquan:
Book Two.

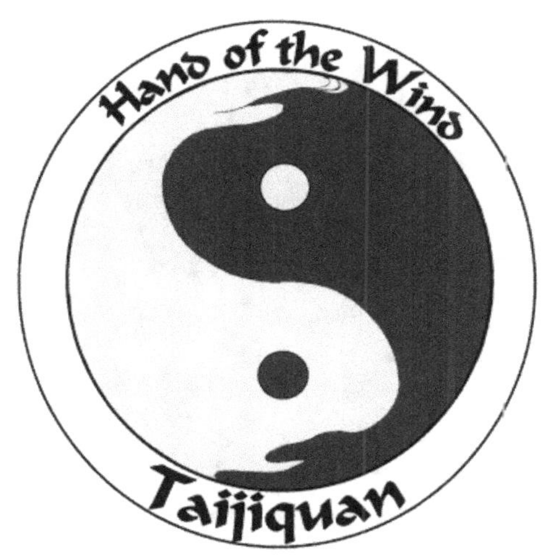

Conrad Robinson

To Console the North Wind

Hand of the Wind Taijiquan:

Book Two.

Taiji Form,
Taiji Feishou Form.

Introduction.

This volume is the second book in a series of three which will detail the full Long Form of the Lee Family style of Tai Chi as I was taught it by my instructors in the 1990s and early 2000s. Like Book One, it is intended to act as an aide-memoire for students of Lee Family Tai Chi – there is no intention for this book to be able to replace good quality 'in-person' teaching. I do not believe that it is possible to learn the movements of the Forms contained herein from a book!

It is my hope that these books will provide a useful reference for students of Hand of the Wind Taijiquan and it is written for them. Students learning the Lee Family style from instructors other than myself may find some things in these volumes that they disagree with – that is fine, we all walk our own path in our study of Tai Chi and we all therefore develop our own understandings. Each person's understanding of Tai Chi should never stop developing and growing and therefore any book on the subject can only ever provide a 'snapshot' of a moment in an individual's journey. I have been very fortunate to share my journey with some remarkable instructors and fantastic students and this book is dedicated to all of them.

Conrad Robinson, 2021

Contents:

Section One: Principles   p6
   Stepping   p7
   Circular Stepping   p10
   The Role of the Spine   p11
   The Three Tantiens   p14

Section Two: Taiji Form   p17

Section Three: Taiji Feishou Form p69

Section One.

Principles.

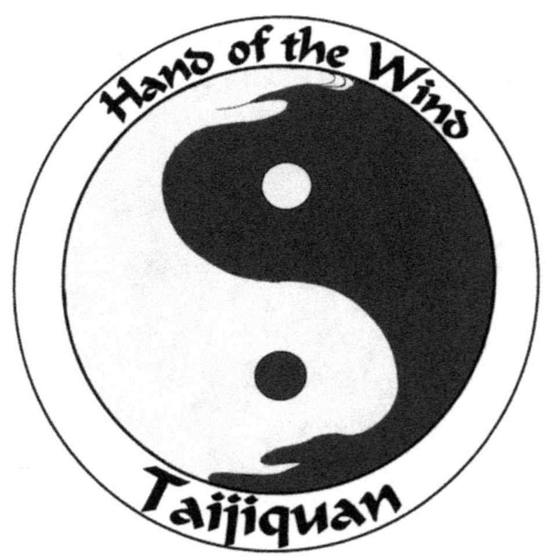

<u>Stepping in the Tai Chi Form.</u>

One of the key aspects of Tai Chi is transitioning from one stance to another and this will often require the movement of a foot. It is vital that these stepping movements are performed correctly if the student wishes to develop their Tai Chi to its full potential.

In order to understand the various stepping movements contained within the Tai Chi Forms, it is important to consider the following question: Why are you stepping?

Often within everyday life, the answer to this question is simply to move from one place to another but this is not the reason for stepping within the Forms. From a martial context there are three reasons why we might wish to step and these are: to evade an attack, to press an attack (whether a strike, kick or throw) or to move into a better position to be able to either attack or defend. Movement is therefore never random but always considered and only performed when necessary – to lift and move a foot is always going to put me at a potential disadvantage from a martial perspective so I do not want to do it for no good reason.

It is therefore necessary to consider the reasons behind each stepping movement within the Forms in order to understand the correct way to perform each of these steps. An examination of the martial application of each movement should point you in the right direction, but also consider other potential applications. For example, the usual application of movement number six of the Tai Chi Form is a throw, but if we consider how that same 'Rotary Dragon' step can also teach us how to perform an outwards back heel kick (similar to Foot Pattern number Sixteen from the Feng Shou syllabus), then we can start to understand the subtleties of how we need to open the hip to perform the step correctly.

It is also vital that we consider the principles of Tai Chi training whenever we think about stepping – particularly the principle of relaxed movement. In order to maintain relaxation whilst stepping it is vital that we do not over-commit to a stance or allow the stance to become rigid (particularly in the knees and the hips).

Re-examining your stances will always be a worthwhile exercise for any student of Tai Chi, however experienced. Pay particular attention to the relaxation of the muscles around the hips and pelvis to allow the 'softening' of the tailbone under the body. The alignment of the coccyx is usually simply described as 'tucking the tailbone under the body' but this often leads to excess tension in the abdomen – instead you should focus on the relaxation of the muscles around the pelvic girdle and allow the tailbone to take up its natural relaxed position which is indeed 'tucked under' the body.

In order for the tailbone to be correctly aligned, it is useful to practice each stance ensuring correct weight distribution into the ball of each foot and finding the correct alignment of the knees. Each foot contains numerous joints and muscles and therefore has the potential to hold a great deal of tension. It is important to work on relaxing the foot and this will allow you to feel the ground beneath you better which will help with balance and controlled stepping. Feet should feel relaxed and 'soft' at all times and it is therefore important to choose footwear for practicing Tai Chi carefully – many shoes (and particularly trainers) have very stiff soles which prevent you from using the feet correctly. Soft rubber soled plimsoles or specialist martial arts shoes are best if you choose to wear shoes at all! Definitely try to avoid the stiff plastic soled plimsoles that are often sold as 'Kung Fu slippers'.

The depth of stances is often a matter of debate within martial arts circles and this is no less true amongst Tai Chi practitioners. If the stance is too 'deep' then it will put excessive pressure onto the knees and prevent the relaxation of the muscles of the legs. If a stance is too shallow it will not be as effective in encouraging Qi to flow to improve health and, martially, our Forms will lack power. There is a certain amount of personal preference involved with finding your preferred depth of stance - just be sure to adhere to all of the principles of Tai Chi training. For the martial students it is very important to train a range of depth of stances because in the fluid situation of combat you will need to be adaptable.

Once you have found your correct stance through practice, it is necessary to learn how to transition from one stance to another without creating unnecessary tensions. Initially, practice stepping into the same stance in all directions (forwards, backwards, left, right and turning both forwards and backwards). As you step, be aware of the transitional stances that you pass through in order to reach the next stance. When you can comfortably step in all directions into the same stance, then you need to learn to step from each stance into every other stance – this will take some time as there are many combinations!

Ensure that your practice of stances is reflected in your practice of the Tai Chi Forms – often people will practice stances but then rely on 'habit' as soon as they start practicing Forms. As you make adjustments to stances to adapt to the changing state of your body (some changes will happen due to natural ageing and some will happen due to the relaxation and softening of your body from your Tai Chi training!) then it is important that those adjustments are carried through into your Tai Chi Forms.

<u>Circular Stepping.</u>

A common feature of stepping in most martial arts is the use of the 'circular step' and Tai Chi is no exception – all of your stepping movements should follow a circular path. Most commonly, an inward circle is used. So, for example, if stepping from a Bear stance forwards into a Dragon stance, then the stepping foot will circle inwards towards the 'centre-line' before continuing the circle outwards again to reach its intended position.

There are times, however, when an outward circle is used – often when 'sweeping' the leg to the side or 'hooking' the foot around an opponent's leg or foot.

In both inward and outward circular stepping, it is the circular movement that allows the step to remain relaxed throughout the step. Be aware of how the hip joint opens and closes during each step.

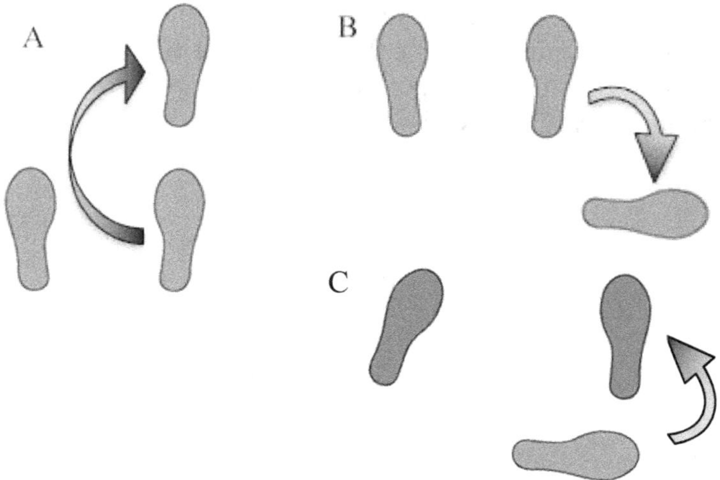

Figure A: An inward circular step forwards from Bear.
Figure B: An outward circular (sweeping) step to the side.
Figure C: An outward circular (hooking) step to the front, from Duck/Monkey to Leopard.
(Note that second foot corrections are not shown.)

<u>The role of the Spine in Tai Chi.</u>

It is still quite common to see people practicing Tai Chi with an unnaturally straight and upright spine – this is very hard to understand in a practice which is intended to be relaxed. To hold the spine upright throughout a Tai Chi Form will build tension in the back, the abdomen and around the hips – all of which prevent 'good' Tai Chi.

To use the spine correctly it is first necessary to provide the proper foundation for the spine. This requires effective stances and the relaxation of the muscles around the pelvis to allow the coccyx to naturally tuck underneath the body and therefore align the sacrum correctly. Once the sacrum is in the correct place the spine can rest on top of it with the shape of each vertebra and the ligaments that hold them together being allowed to shape the spine correctly. It is therefore vital that excess tension in the back, the abdomen and the chest is not pulling the spine out of shape.

When the spine is allowed to adopt its natural shape, it will allow the whole upper body to relax into its correct posture and the resulting relaxation will make the whole body feel softer and more 'fluid'. This in turn will allow the spine to move more as the joints between the vertebrae are loosened, taking the pressure off the discs and freeing any nerves that are being compressed.

Within the Tai Chi Form the spine does move, consider the opening of the thoracic spine within movement number two or the twisting movement through the spine of movement number fifteen, and it is vital that we learn to feel and understand these movements and their affect on the spine and the rest of the body.

A sequence of the Form that is often used to encourage movement within the spine is the 'Fair Lady Weaving' sequence encompassing movements eight to eleven. Initially, a relatively 'physical' interpretation of these movements is often taught to beginners where they are taught to move their hands forwards 'over the ball' in move eight, coming back under the ball in move nine before reversing those circles for movements ten and eleven. This tends to lead to excessive movement of the shoulders and arms and so it is important that as students progress, they are taught to use the body to move the arms more. Part of this comes from the regular opening and closing of the chest and body which occurs throughout the Form but the real core of this sequence lies in the movement of the spine.

At the end of movement number seven the head is 'rolled' over to look down and this movement is generated within the thoracic spine (so the upper part of the back – not the neck!). As you start move number eight you straighten the upper spine and this brings the hands up to shoulder height (the simultaneous opening of the chest aligns the hands correctly). As you then move forwards into Dragon stance, there is a feeling of the pelvis moving forwards fractionally before the shoulders – this creates the 'over the ball' feeling without having to move the arms or shoulders. In move number nine, as you shift back to Monkey stance there is the same feeling of 'hips before shoulders'. At the end of move nine, the chest opens and turns the hands before moving forwards into Dragon again in move ten – this time with the shoulders leading the pelvis slightly.

This idea of 'hips before shoulders' and then 'shoulders before hips' is of course a transitional stage within our development of the Tai Chi Form – we are using gross physical movement (although it may be too subtle for many observers to notice) to learn how the movements should feel. We then need to internalize the movements more and we can do this by thinking about moving the lower and middle Tantiens rather than the hips and shoulders. Ultimately, what we are trying to achieve within this sequence is to master the technique referred to as the 'spine whip'.

The 'spine whip' is a term that we use to refer to movements where either the upper or lower portion of the spine moves before the other and then there is a 'whip-like' movement through the spine as the other section of the spine catches up. This is used within the martial arts to provide power into striking techniques and within the health side of the art encourages the loose natural movement of the spine encouraging Qi flow as well as taking pressure off the intravertebral discs and the nerves that exit and enter the spine along its length. To assist with the execution of this 'whipping' movement of the spine (remember that it is usually performed slowly and not quickly as the term 'whipping' may imply!) it is useful to be aware of the alignment of the sacrum and utilise the relaxation of the 'Kua' to allow the pelvis to adjust as necessary for each movement – this is an area where expert tuition is advised to ensure that the stances do not become corrupted by adjustment of the pelvis.

<u>The Three Tantiens and their role in Tai Chi.</u>

Within Qigong theory it is common to refer to the Three Tantiens and these are described as 'centres' of Qi within the body that are often said to relate to different aspects of our being. The Lower Tantien is the one that is most often referred to in Tai Chi training and is said to reside below the navel in the centre of the body (so just in front of the spine) and this is usually considered to be the most 'grounded' and physical of the Tantiens. The Middle Tantien is located in the centre of the chest (so occupying the same space as the Heart organ) and is usually linked to the more emotional aspects of life. The Upper Tantien is located above and between the eyes, back into the centre of the skull and is often related to spiritual practices.

The Lower Tantien is referred to the most by the majority of Tai Chi Teachers. The Upper Tantien is often effectively ignored in much Tai Chi training and the Middle Tantien is often only rarely referred to by most teachers. The full use and development of the Three Tantiens within Qigong training is well beyond the scope of this book but some understanding is useful for Tai Chi Practitioners.

Within Qigong practice the Lower Tantien is often described as a 'pool' of Qi and is described as being warm so analogies with a 'swamp' are commonly used. In accordance with Qigong theory relating to the Triple Burner or Triple Warmer the Lower Tantien is where Qi sinks to and is then heated before rising further up through the body (often described as 'mist-like' as it rises).

The Qi in the Middle Tantien is therefore considered to have a more rarefied quality than the Qi in the Lower Tantien. It is also said to be cooler and the Qi then cools further and becomes even more ethereal as it rises to the Upper Tantien.

Some Tai Chi teachers describe a single Tantien for the purposes of Tai Chi training and they sometimes describe this as a 'ball' that occupies the lower half of the torso (so encompassing the Lower Tantien and extending up to the Middle Tantien). Whilst this can be a useful simplification of the full Tantien theory, it is my

14

feeling that to get a full understanding of the uses of the Tantien in Tai Chi practice, then this is too much of an over-simplification.

From our Qigong practice we aim to develop an awareness of the Qi in the Lower Tantien and to draw Qi down into the 'pool' at Lower Tantien where it is heated and then initiates movement. This sense of movement beginning within the Lower Tantien is necessary to be able to initiate the movement of the Tai Chi Form and to implement martial techniques.

Within Tai Chi practice, we are said to draw power from the ground through the legs and then to direct this power from the Tantien. The movements of the Short Form of Lee Family Style Tai Chi are directed through the Lower Tantien, but as you extend your practice into the Long Form and learn the movements described in this volume you will notice a change in the character of the Form. As you progress into the movements beyond number Fifty, there is a shift to directing movements through the Middle Tantien and then farther into the Form the emphasis shifts up and down between Lower and Middle Tantien. It is clear, then, why some teachers would choose to simplify the idea of the Tantiens to use a single focus that takes in both the Lower and Middle Tantiens. However, it is the study of the interactions between both of these Tantiens that can help us to unlock more of the deeper aspects of our Internal practice.

Aim to be aware of the area between the Lower and Middle Tantiens as you practice your Tai Chi movements. It is particularly important to consider this area and the physical and energetic changes within it as you practice the 'Eight Energies' within the Tai Chi movements. As you practice movements relating to each of the 'Eight Energies', be conscious of the interactions between Lower and Middle Tantien and then utilize that awareness to power the 'Eight Energies' by initiating those same interactions – following the idea of practicing a movement more physically to feel how it affects the body and then 'turning it around' to create the effect within the body in order to initiate the movement. This is a key step in moving your Tai Chi practice from an external, physical exercise to a truly 'Internal' practice.

The sense of directing movement from the Middle Tantien in some movements rather than from the Lower Tantien leads to a more expansive feel to the moves and is also integral to our practice of the Feishou Form. When practicing the Feishou Form there is a strong connection to the ground through the Bubbling Spring points in the soles of the feet. Try to cultivate the feeling of almost 'pushing' through the Bubbling Spring points to power the movements and then utilize the Middle Tantien to control and direct the movements. This leads to the more expansive feel of the Feishou Form and explains why many teachers refer to it as the 'Tai Chi Dance'.

The understanding and ability of how to direct movement through either the Lower Tantien or Middle Tantien is particularly important to students of the martial aspects of Tai Chi. Directing through Lower Tantien leads to a good basic level of martial skill but it is when you can use either Lower or Middle Tantiens that you start to truly appreciate the subtleties of Tai Chi as a martial art.

It is, of course, vital that you maintain the 'groundedness' of your Tai Chi practice even as you learn to direct movement through the Middle Tantien and this is an area where practice of the Feishou Form alongside the Tai Chi Form can provide great advances in your understanding and skill level.

Section Two.

The Taiji Form.

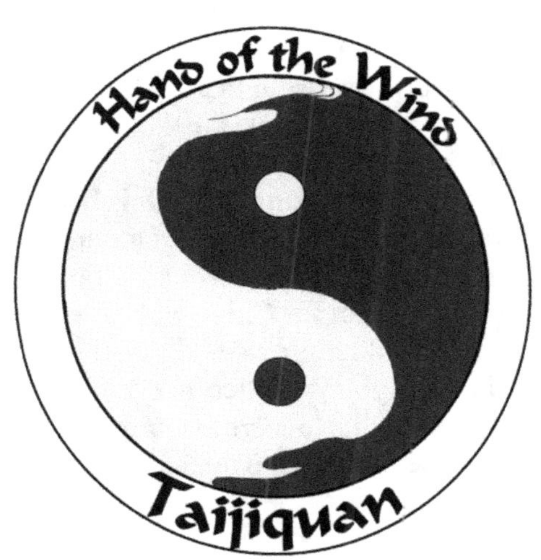

The Taiji Form.

Movements 51 to 95.

Book One 'To the Edge of the Cyclone' detailed the movements of the first fifteen sequences of the Lee Family Tai Chi Form as taught in Hand of the Wind Taijiquan classes. This volume covers the next fourteen sequences and two of the movements from sequence number thirty 'Consoling the North Wind'. I have chosen to cover up to movement number ninety-five in this book as it provides a good posture to finish on and it conveniently breaks up the remainder of the one hundred and forty movement Form into evenly sized 'chunks' – Book Three will detail the remaining movements of the Form.

It is worth stressing that it is not really possible to learn these movements from a book but hopefully this volume can help to refresh memories and assist you in your practice of the Tai Chi Form. If you are making use of this book, it is likely that you have been training for a considerable amount of time and are fully aware of the importance of the Form as a tool and not to view it as some sort of goal. Your Tai Chi Form should be constantly evolving as your understanding grows and as your body softens and re-shapes itself through your practice of Tai Chi. Aim to take all of the lessons that you have learnt from your practice of the Short Form and apply them to the movements described herein.

On the following pages there is a quick reference table of the movements described in this section, similar to the one provided in Book One.

Sequence	Move	Stance	Facing
The Edge of the Cyclone	47	Left Monkey	South
	48	Right Dragon	"
	49	Right Cat	"
	50	Right Dragon	"
Single Whip Unleashed	51	Left Duck	"
	52	Left Dragon	West
The Double Whip	53	Left Cat	"
	54	Left Leopard	South
The Playful Dog	55	Left Cat	East
	56	Left Dragon	"
	57	Left Dog	"
	58	Left Dragon	"
Catching Chickens	59	Right Monkey	South
	60	Left Dragon	"
	61	Left Leopard	"
	62	Right Dragon	"
The Archer Prepares	63	Riding Horse	East
	64	Right Dragon	"
	65	Right Cat	"
Mount the Wild Horse	66	Right Dog	"
	67	Riding Horse	South
	68	Left Dragon	East
	69	Left Cat	"
Flexing of the Single Whip	70	Right Dragon	West
	71	Left Cat	East
	72	Left Dragon	"

Sequence	Move	Stance	Facing
Repulse the Monkey	73	Right Leopard	South
	74	Left Dragon	··
	75	Left Cat	··
	76	Left Dragon	East
Grasp the Bird's Tail	77	Left Cat	··
	78	Right Dragon	West
The Crane Raises its Head	79	Right Monkey	··
	80	Right Crane	··
Roll and Stretch	81	Left Cat	South
	82	Left Dragon	··
The Five Elements	83	Riding Horse	East
	84	Left Dragon	··
	85	Left Cat	··
	86	Left Leopard	South
	87	Right Monkey	West
The Double Whip	88	Right Leopard	South
	89	Left Cat	East
Waving the Hands in the Clouds	90	Left Dog	··
	91	Right Duck	··
	92	Left Dragon	··
	93	Left Snake	··
Consoling the North Wind	94	Right Dragon	South
	95	Riding Horse	··
Gather Earth's Energy	(1)	Eagle	··
	(2)	Eagle	··
	(3)	Eagle	··

Within this section each movement of the Form is presented with photographs of the end position. Photographs are provided from the 'front' and from one side for each position – the larger photo is from the perspective of a viewer standing to the front at the start of the form; and the smaller image shows the view from the side on which that picture is presented. There is also a description of the movement required to reach that position: this is broken down into stance movement, posture movement and sometimes notes on timing.

Although the movements are separated into stance and posture for convenience within this book, remember that the stance and posture work together and the movements of both the lower and upper bodies must be coordinated correctly as described in the timing notes or often within the description of the posture movement. The separation of the stance and posture movements in this volume is intended to reinforce the idea that it is often good to practice the movement of the stance first and then to add the posture movement on afterwards.

As in Book One, the preceding table and the descriptions of the movements refer to compass directions. These are for reference only! Although the descriptions assume that you are facing South when you begin the Form, it really does not matter which direction you are facing. The compass directions are simply a convenient means to say that certain movements are facing the same way as you began the Form and some are facing ninety degrees to the left (given as East) or ninety degrees to the right (given as West)!

Move 50.

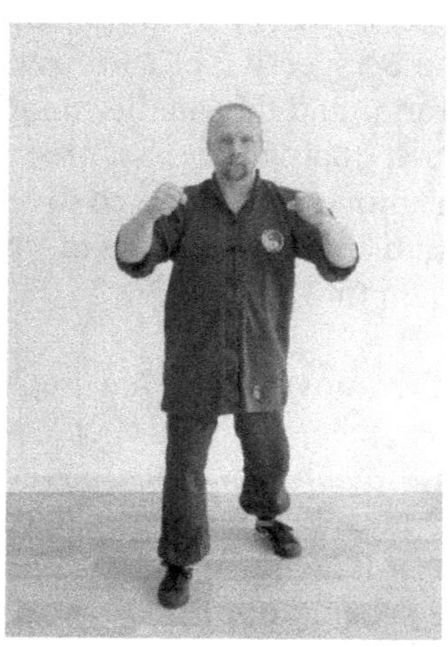

Stance: Right Dragon
Facing: South

At the end of the Short Form (as covered in 'To the Edge of the Cyclone'/Book One) we finish in a Right Dragon Stance facing South with the hands in soft fists extended in front of the Shoulders.

No description of this movement is provided here as it is covered in Book One.

The Form continues from this position into Move 51 as follows.

Move 51.

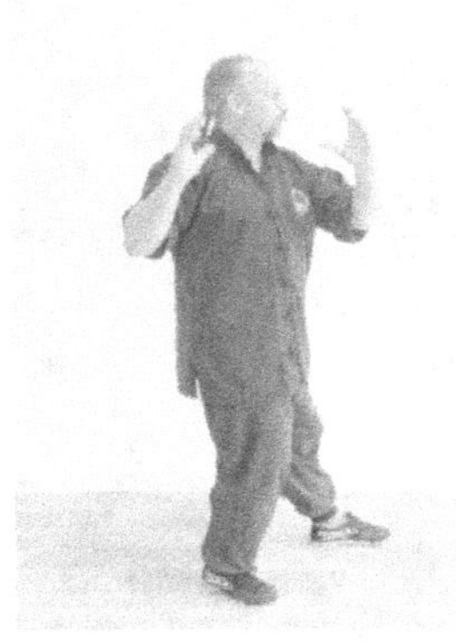 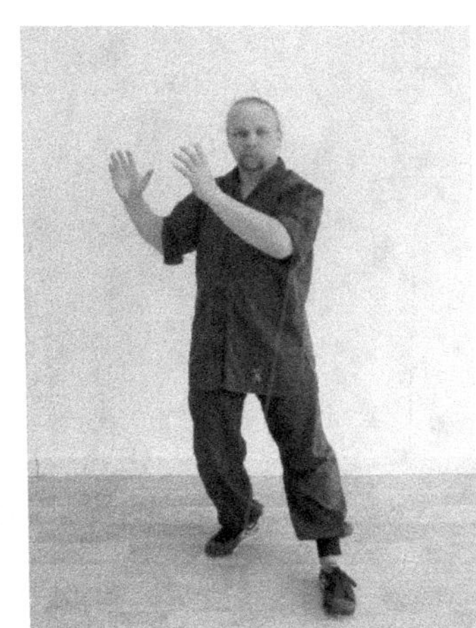

Stance: Left Duck
Facing: South

Stance movement:

The weight shifts back onto the left leg (so into a Right Duck stance). Then step the right foot back and shift the weight backwards to come into a Left Duck stance, straightening the left foot at the end of the movement.

Posture movement:

The body rolls very slightly to the right as the left hand comes on top and the right hand moves below as if holding a 'ball'. Draw the hands (holding the 'ball') back and down beside the right hip before raising and rotating the ball to shoulder height ('ball' held horizontally with the left hand in front) and the upper body turned to the right (head still looking forwards).

Timing:

Step the right foot backwards when the 'ball' is beside the right hip.

Move 52.

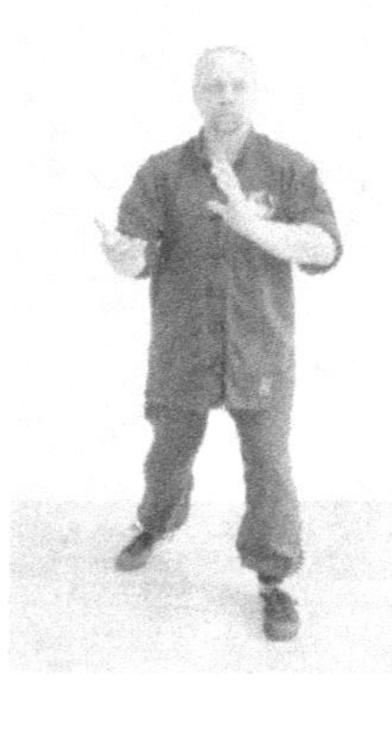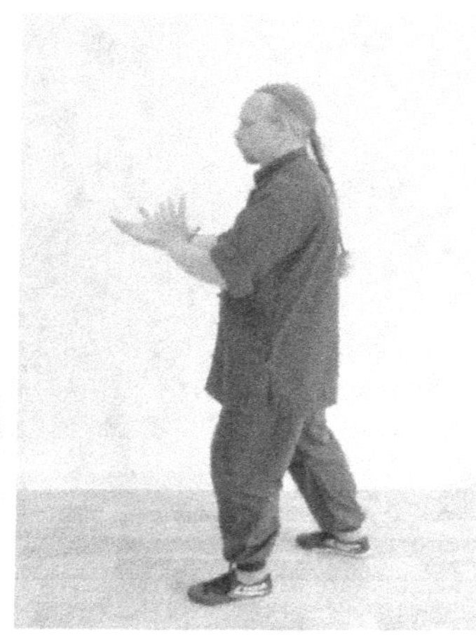

Stance: Left Dragon
Facing: West

<u>Stance movement:</u>

Step the left foot across the front of the standing leg, placing the foot into position and then shifting the weight onto the left leg and correcting the right foot (heel-toe) to finish in a Left Dragon stance turned ninety degrees to the right.

<u>Posture movement:</u>

The right hand turns palm downwards and rolls across the body to under the left elbow (straightening the waist and collapsing the chest). Open the chest to bring the right arm out from under the left in a horizontal motion with the elbow and forearm leading. Meanwhile, the left hand comes down to rest in front of the chest on its own side of the centre-line.

<u>Timing:</u>

The waist straightens and the right hand comes underneath the left elbow before stepping the left foot. Open the chest as the weight shifts into the Dragon stance.

Move 53.

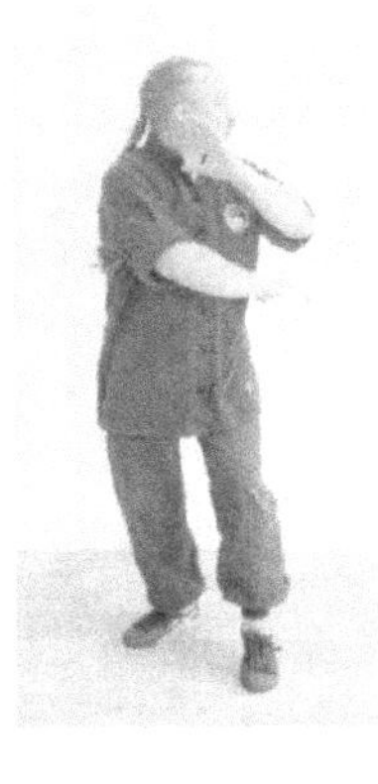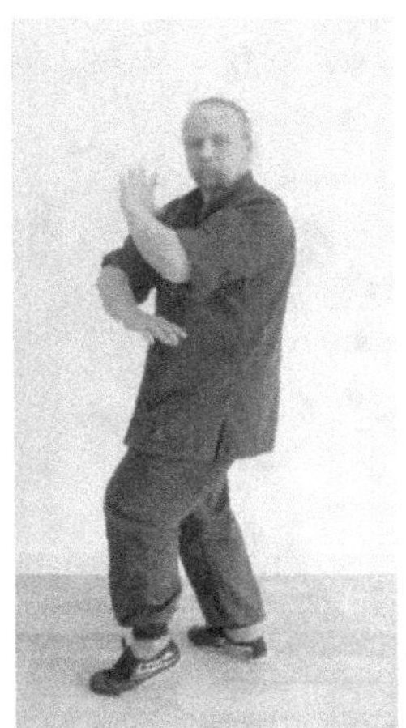

Stance: Left Cat
Facing: West

<u>Stance movement:</u>

Draw the weight back onto the right leg and bring the left foot into position for Left Cat stance.

<u>Posture movement:</u>

Open the chest to separate the hands, then the right hand rolls over to palm down. The chest then closes bringing the right hand underneath the left elbow and the left hand to in front of the right shoulder. The waist turns slightly to the left and the head turns further to the left to look over the left shoulder.

<u>Timing:</u>

Open the chest whilst still in Dragon, then draw back into Cat as the right hand moves under the left arm, turn the waist and head as you settle into Cat stance.

Move 54.

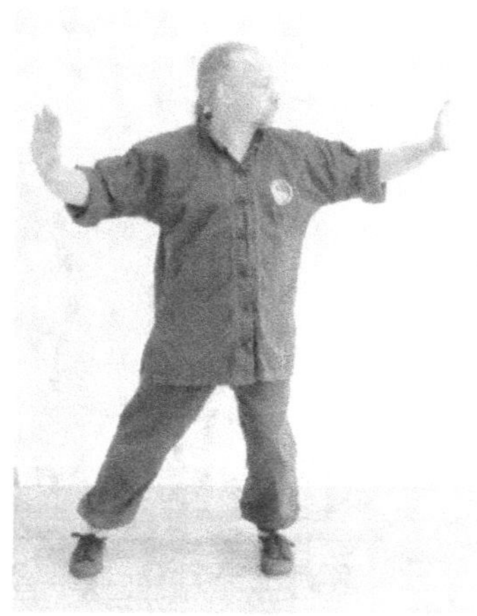

Stance: Left Leopard
Facing: South

<u>Stance movement:</u>

Step the left foot behind you so that your heels are in line with each other, pointing the toes to the South. Then, bring the weight onto the left foot as you turn to face South into Left Leopard (correcting the right foot at the end of the movement).

<u>Posture movement:</u>

The hands open outwards at chest height until they are extended to the sides at shoulder level with the palms of the hands facing away from the body. Turn the head to look at the left hand.

<u>Timing:</u>

Place the left foot first as the hands start to open outwards. The hands continue outwards as you turn and then turn the head and correct the right foot at the end of the movement.

Move 55.

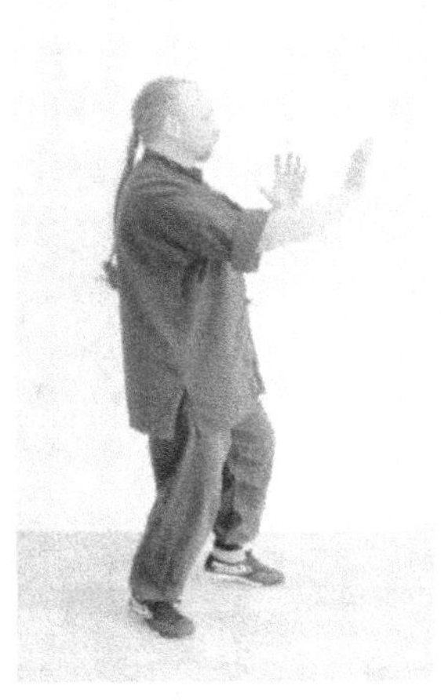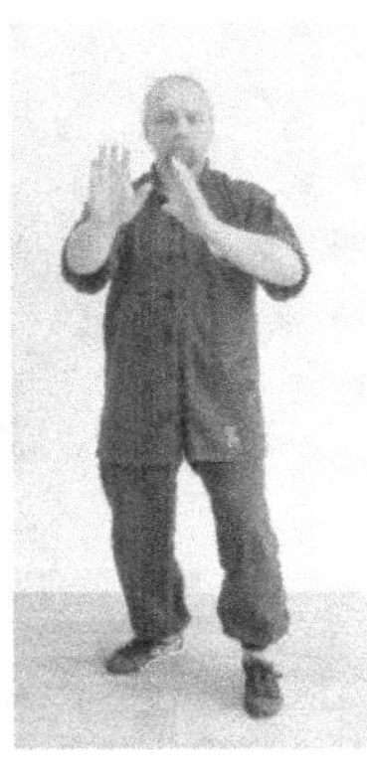

Stance: Left Cat
Facing: East

<u>Stance movement:</u>

Shift the weight onto the left leg and correct the right foot around forty-five degrees to the right. Bring the weight back onto the right foot, turning the body to the left to face East and then draw the left foot back into a Cat stance.

<u>Posture movement:</u>

The right hand swings around at shoulder height until extended to the front of the body in line with the right shoulder (the palm facing away from the body). The left hand moves inwards to settle in place in front of the chest on its own side of the centre-line.

<u>Timing:</u>

The right arm initially moves with the body as the body turns and then continues to swing inwards as the weight settles into the Cat stance.

Move 56.

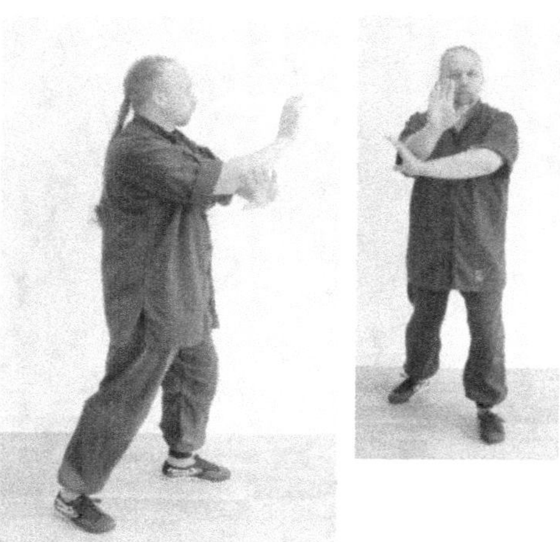

Stance: Left Dragon
Facing: East

<u>Stance movement:</u>

Step the left foot forwards and then bring the weight forwards to come into a Dragon stance.

<u>Posture movement:</u>

Open the chest and turn the waist approximately forty-five degrees to the right so that the hands come to holding a 'ball' in front of the chest. As you come into the Dragon stance, the waist straightens bringing the right hand forwards in a 'push'. The left shoulder 'collapses' inwards so that the left hand is on the outside of the right arm as it pushes forwards.

<u>Timing:</u>

The turn of the waist to the right and opening of the chest to hold the 'ball' should happen whilst still in Cat stance.

Move 57.

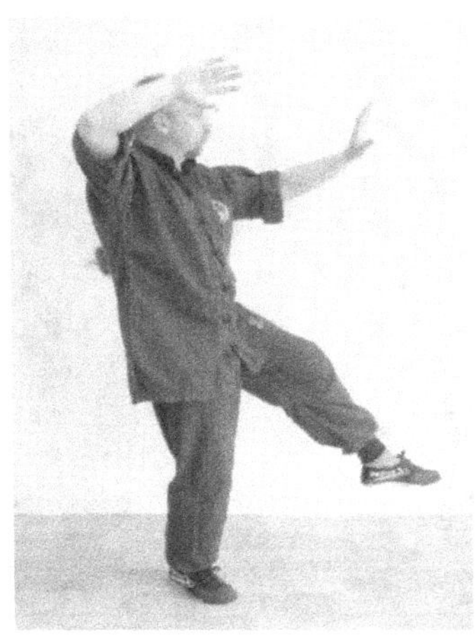

Stance: Left Dog
Facing: East

<u>Stance movement:</u>

Draw the weight back onto the right leg and lift the left leg up into a Dog stance, still facing East.

<u>Posture movement:</u>

Roll the right elbow outwards and upwards (so that the fingers are pointing forwards with the thumb edge facing downwards) before drawing the elbow back past the right side of the head, turning the shoulders approximately forty-five degrees to your right. The left hand extends out and forwards to finish with the palm facing forwards in front of the left shoulder.

Move 58.

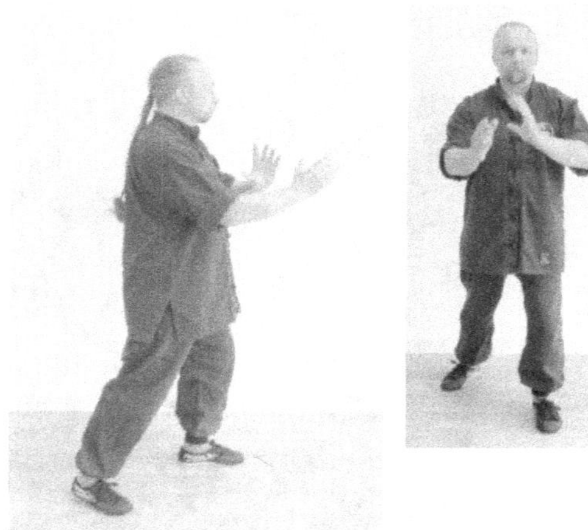

Stance: Left Dragon
Facing: East

<u>Stance movement:</u>

Place the left foot back down to the front of the body and shift the weight forwards into a Dragon stance.

<u>Posture movement:</u>

The right hand presses downwards on the right side of the body until it is beside the right hip, it then continues to circle upwards and to the front, turning the hand so that the fingers are pointing forwards with the little finger edge downwards. The right hand finishes its circle by 'spear-ing' upwards to sternum height. The left hand draws inwards to rest in front of the chest on its own side of the centre-line.

<u>Timing:</u>

Place the foot as the right hand presses down and then shift the weight forwards as the right hand spears forwards and upwards.

Move 59.

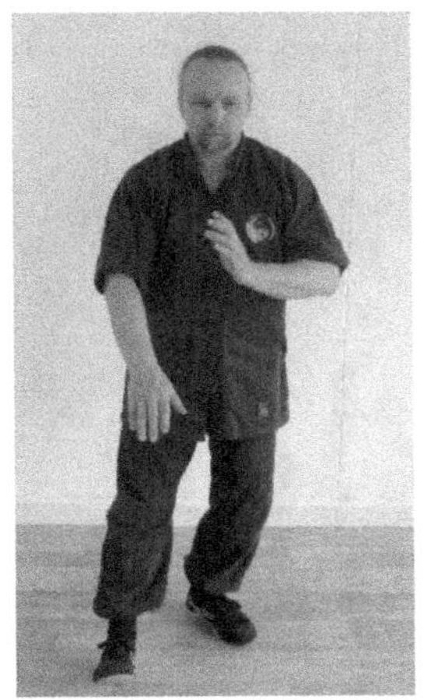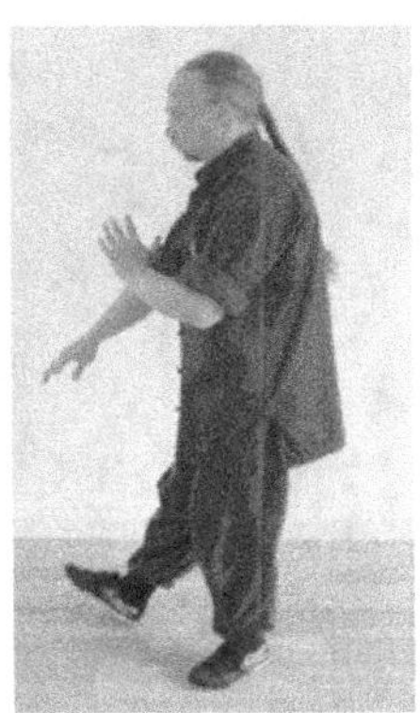

Stance: Right Monkey
Facing: South

Stance movement:

The weight shifts back onto the right foot turning the body to face South. The left foot then steps behind the body and the weight shifts back onto it, lifting the toes of the front foot to finish in Monkey stance facing South.

Posture movement:

Turn the right hand to palm upwards then allow the arm to lead as the body turns to the right to face South. The right hand then turns palm down and 'pats' down towards the right knee.

Timing:

First, turn the right hand palm upwards. Then, turn the body to the right before stepping the left foot back as the right hand turns to palm downwards. Settle the weight into the Monkey stance as the right hand 'pats' down.

Move 60.

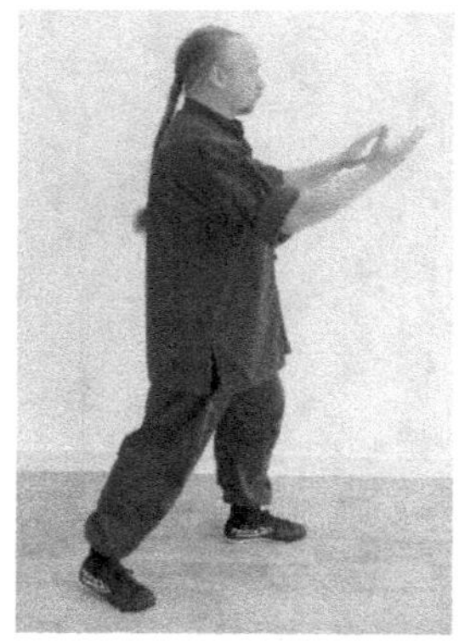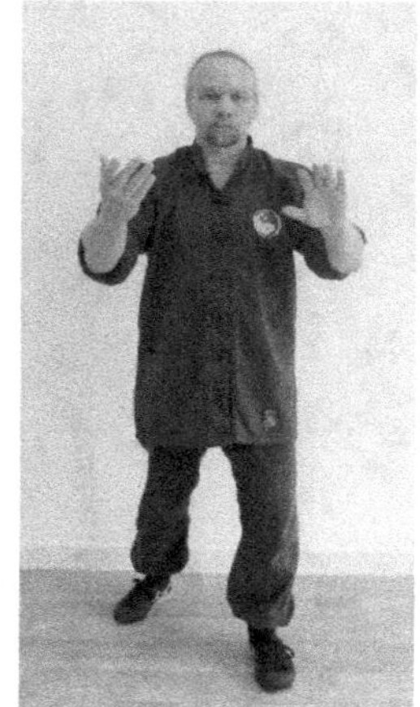

Stance: Left Dragon
Facing: South

<u>Stance movement:</u>

Correct the right foot outwards onto an angle to the right (in readiness to step into Left Dragon). Shift the weight forwards onto the right foot and then step the left foot through to come into a Left Dragon stance.

<u>Posture movement:</u>

The right hand comes up underneath the left elbow (palm upwards) collapsing the chest. As the chest then opens again, the hands 'scissor' outwards until they are in front of the shoulders (left hand palm down and right hand palm up).

<u>Timing:</u>

Correct the right foot and shift the weight onto it as the right hand comes underneath the left elbow. Step through and bring the weight forwards as the hands 'scissor' outwards.

Move 61.

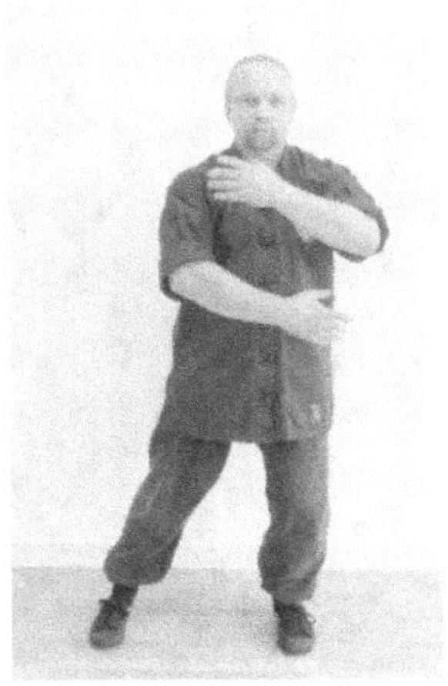

Stance: Left Leopard
Facing: South

<u>Stance movement:</u>

Draw the weight back onto the right leg and then step the left foot back and across to a position in line with the right foot, pointing the toes forwards as you place the foot. The weight then transfers onto the left foot into a Leopard stance, correcting the right foot to parallel at the end of the movement.

<u>Posture movement:</u>

The hands continue to open outwards with the left hand also turning palm upwards. Bring the elbows back towards the hips, before 'wrapping' the arms around into position to 'embrace yourself' (right arm around waist, left hand facing in towards right shoulder).

<u>Timing:</u>

The weight shifts onto the right foot as the arms draw back and down towards hips. Step to the left and shift into Leopard as the arms wrap inwards.

Move 62.

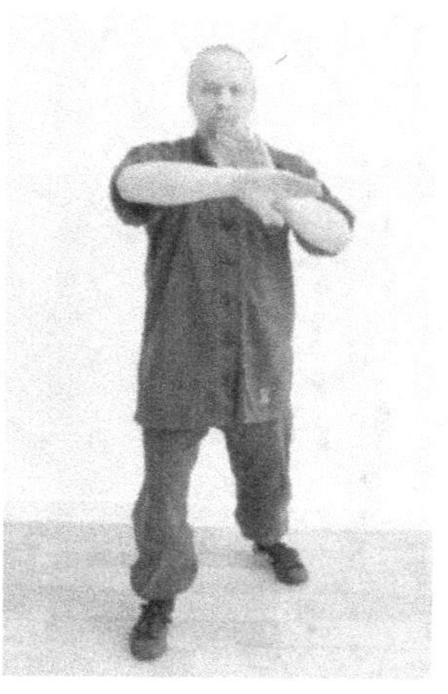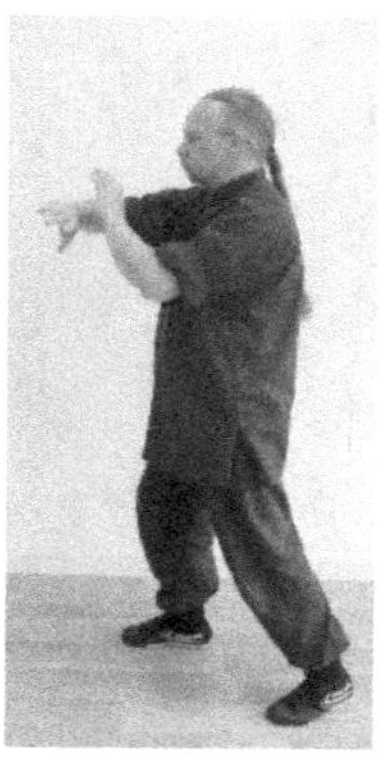

Stance: Right Dragon
Facing: South

<u>Stance movement:</u>

Step the right foot forwards and place into position. Then, shift the weight forwards into the Dragon stance.

<u>Posture movement:</u>

The left hand draws down the right arm and then 'pushes' the right arm up and out to the front. Finish with the right forearm extended to the front with the right hand palm facing down and forwards (on a forty-five degree angle). The left palm is facing towards the right forearm just above the wrist.

Move 63.

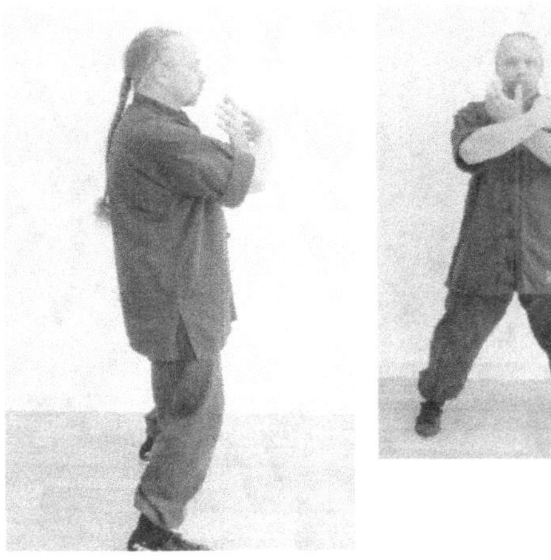

Stance: Riding Horse
Facing: East

<u>Stance movement:</u>

Shift the weight back onto the left foot, turning the upper body to the left as you correct the right foot ninety degrees to the left. Step the left foot back into line with the right foot and settle the weight equally onto both feet into Riding Horse stance.

<u>Posture movement:</u>

The arms open forwards and upwards before circling out and down. They then continue their circles to come up in front of the body with the right arm crossed over the left arm (similar to move number Seventeen).

<u>Timing:</u>

Open the arms up and out as you turn and correct the right foot, continue the circles to finish as you settle into the Riding Horse.

Move 64.

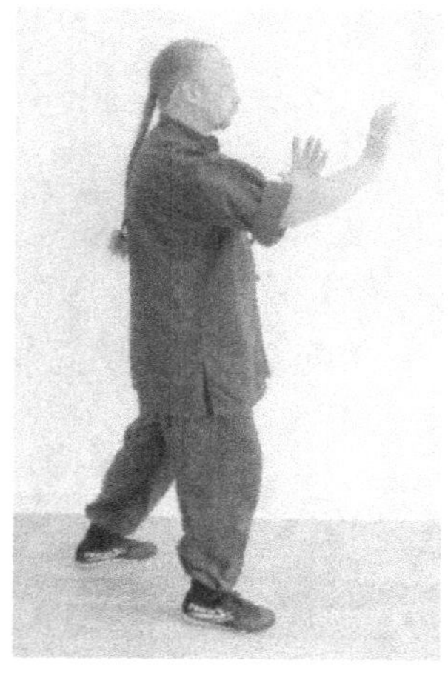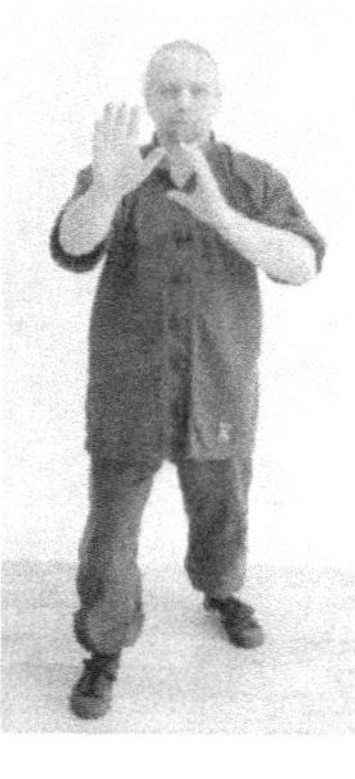

Stance: Right Dragon
Facing: East

<u>Stance movement:</u>

The weight shifts onto the left leg and the right foot steps forwards before transferring the weight forwards into the Dragon stance.

<u>Posture movement:</u>

The hands open out to a 'holding-the-ball' position in front of the chest, turning the waist a little to the left. The left hand settles into position in front of the chest as the right hand 'pushes' forwards and you straighten the waist to bring the shoulders in line with the hips.

<u>Timing:</u>

Form the 'ball' with the hands and turn to the left as the weight shifts onto the left leg. Straighten the body as you come forwards into the Dragon.

Move 65.

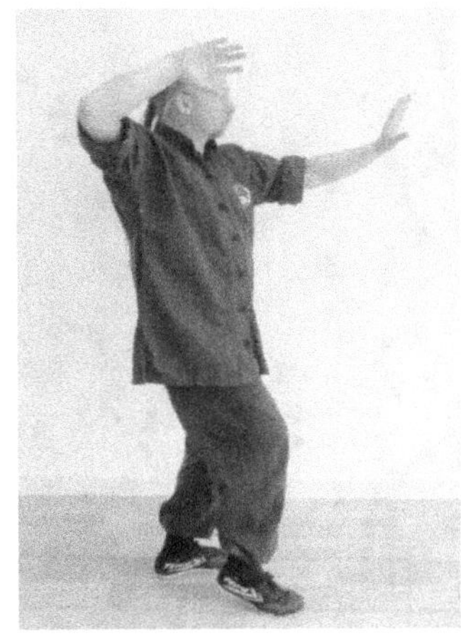 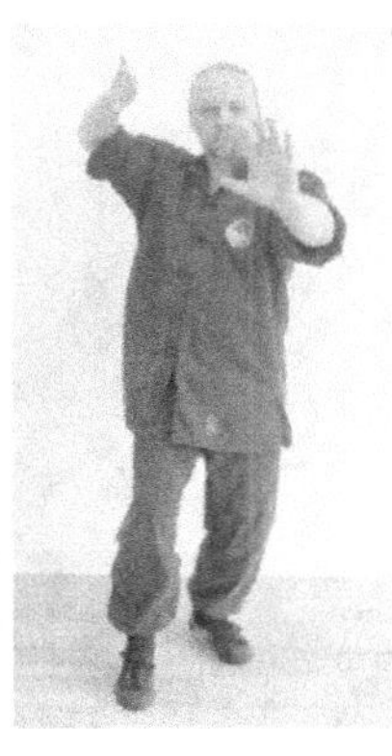

Stance: Right Cat
Facing: East

<u>Stance movement:</u>

The weight shifts back onto the left leg, drawing the right foot back and then lifting the heel into Cat stance.

<u>Posture movement:</u>

Roll the right elbow up and back (opening the chest) as you turn the upper body a little to the right. This brings the left arm forwards into position (turn the palm to face the front) and the right hand faces outwards at head height.

Move 66.

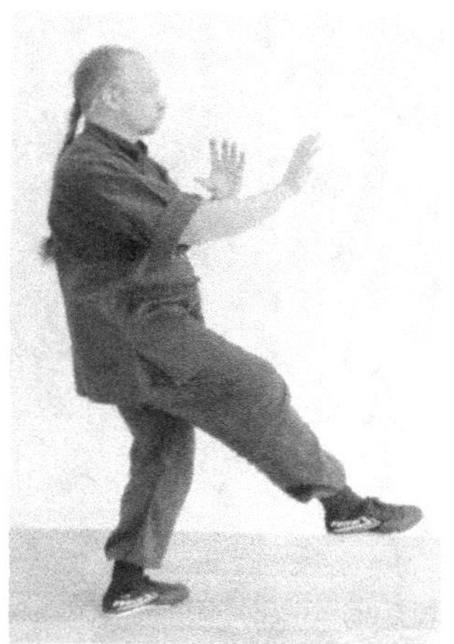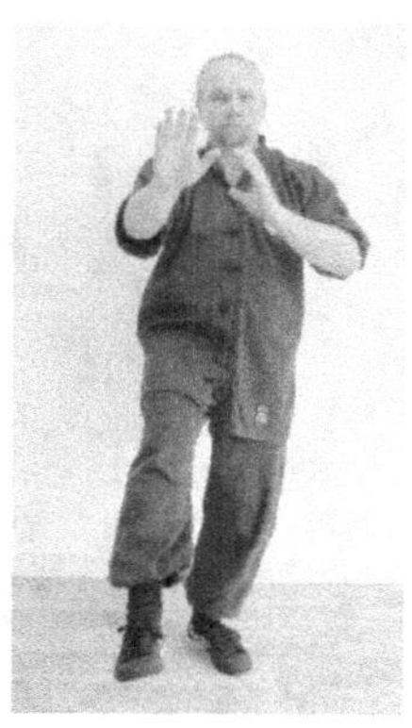

Stance: Right Dog
Facing: East

<u>Stance movement:</u>

The right foot lifts in front of the body into Dog stance.

<u>Posture movement:</u>

The right hand 'presses' down towards the right hip and then comes up (at the same time as the leg) to face palm forwards at shoulder height. The left hand settles into position in front of the chest.

Move 67.

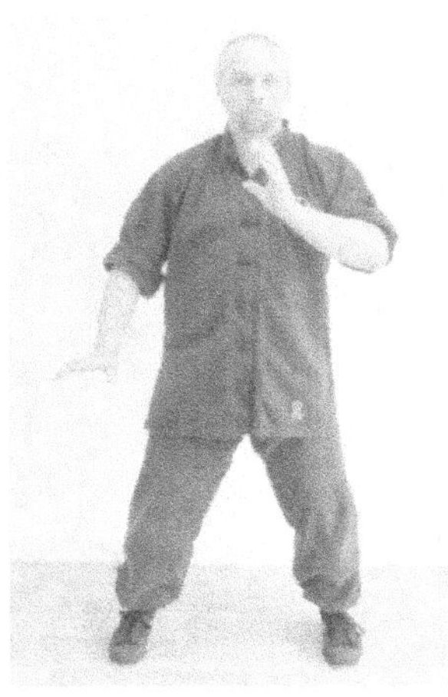

Stance: Riding Horse
Facing: South

<u>Stance movement:</u>

The right leg 'swings' around towards the right to land behind the body, in line with the left foot and with the toes pointing towards the South. Turn the body ninety degrees to the right shifting the weight into the right foot and then correct the left foot into the Riding Horse stance.

<u>Posture movement:</u>

The right hand swings around with the leg to finish palm down beside the right hip. The left hand draws a small circle downwards and outwards before coming back over and in to finish again in front of the chest (this left hand movement coincides with the final shift of the weight and correction of the left foot).

Move 68.

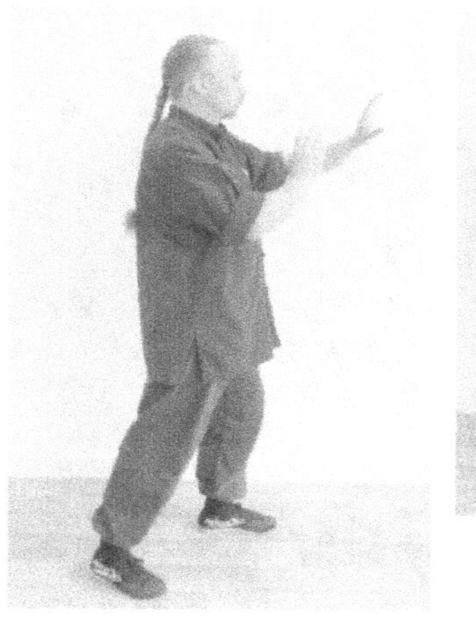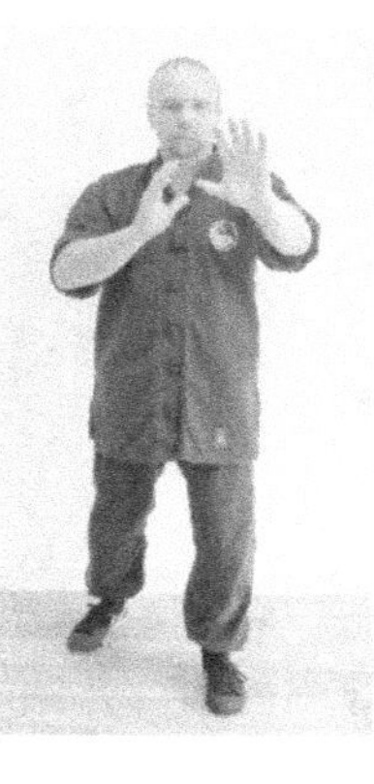

Stance: Left Dragon
Facing: East

<u>Stance movement:</u>

The weight shifts onto the right foot to enable the left foot to step to the left into position for a Dragon stance facing East. Draw the weight onto the left foot, straightening the hips into the Dragon stance and correcting the right foot as you settle into Dragon stance.

<u>Posture movement:</u>

The left hand continues its circle from the end of the previous move before moving out to the left to finish in front of the left shoulder. The right hand follows the left arm up into position in front of the chest.

Move 69.

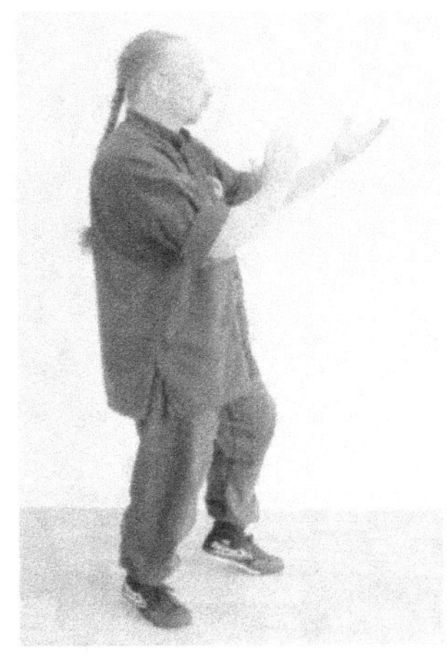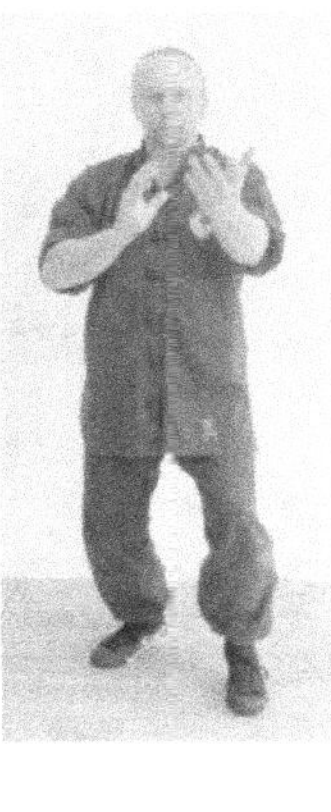

Stance: Left Cat
Facing: East

<u>Stance movement:</u>

Bring the weight back onto the right foot and draw the left foot back into Cat stance.

<u>Posture movement:</u>

The left hand rolls out to the left side and then follows a circle out and down, then in and upwards to finish palm up in front of the left shoulder. The right arm remains in place in front of the chest.

Move 70.

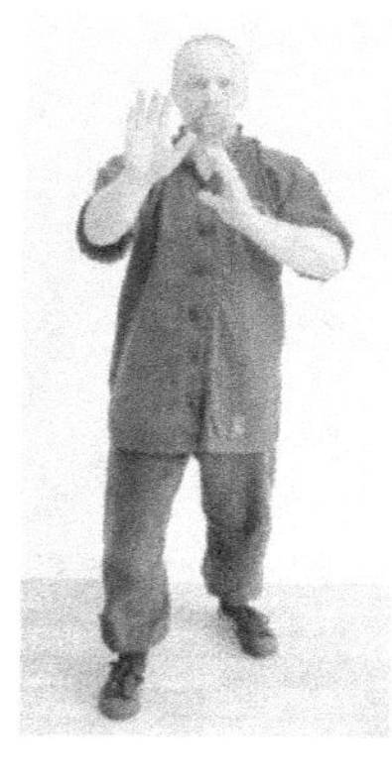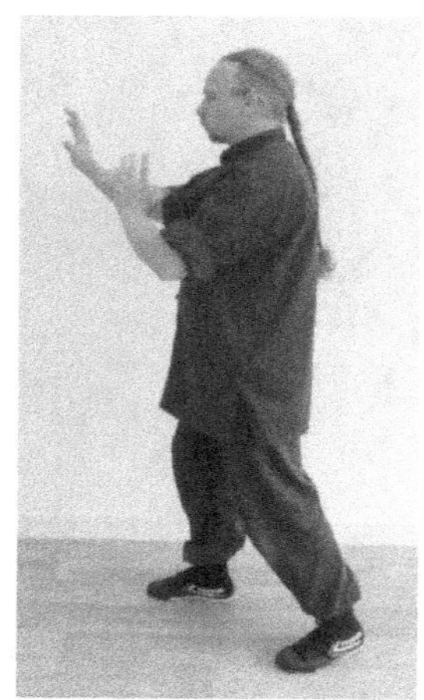

Stance: Right Dragon
Facing: West

<u>Stance movement:</u>

Drop the left heel onto the floor, then pivot the left foot a three-quarter turn to the right (to point South-West). Shift the weight onto the left foot and step the right foot around to place in position for Dragon stance facing West before settling the weight into the Dragon stance.

<u>Posture movement:</u>

The right arm leads outwards as you turn to the right to finish palm forwards in front of the right shoulder. The left hand follows the right arm around to finish in front of the chest.

Move 71.

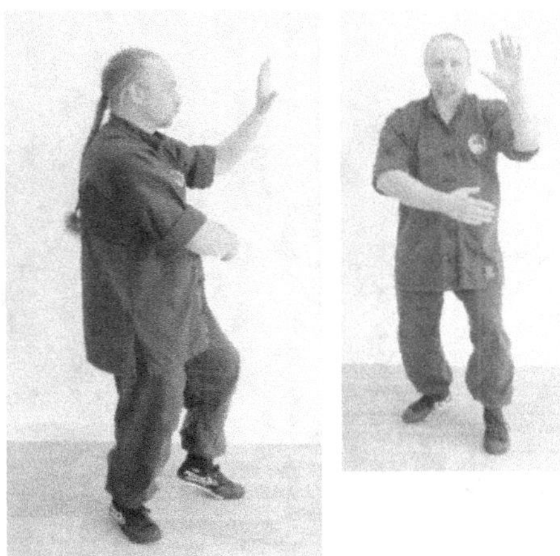

Stance: Left Cat
Facing: East

<u>Stance movement:</u>

The weight shifts back onto the left foot and then correct the right foot around to point towards the South-East. Draw the weight onto the right foot and bring the left foot around as you turn one hundred and eighty degrees to face East, drawing the left foot back into Cat stance.

<u>Posture movement:</u>

The left hand comes around with the body to finish with the palm facing forwards at head height forward from the left shoulder. The right hand sweeps around to face in towards the waist on the left side of the body.

<u>Timing:</u>

Draw the left foot back into Cat as the left hand draws in towards the waist.

Move 72.

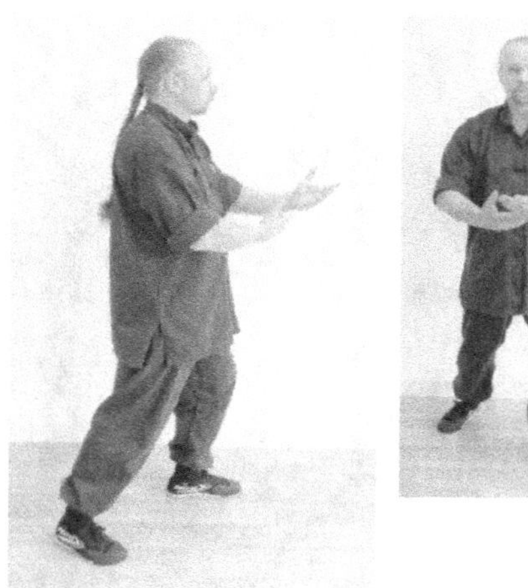

Stance: Left Dragon
Facing: East

<u>Stance movement:</u>

Step the left foot forwards and then move the weight into Dragon stance.

<u>Posture movement:</u>

The left hand 'pats' downwards, followed by the right hand, towards the left knee. The body then turns slightly to the right so that the hands come up in front of the right hip (left hand above right, both palms up). Then open the chest, as the weight shifts forwards and the waist straightens, so that the hands open outwards to finish with the right fingers pointing towards the left wrist (so, very much like doing movement number four on the opposite side).

Move 73.

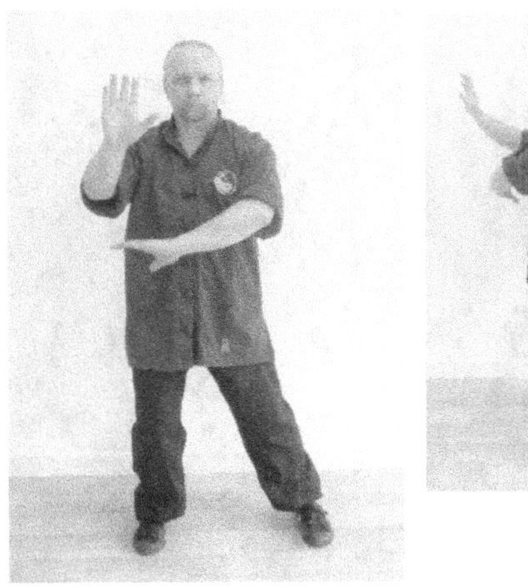
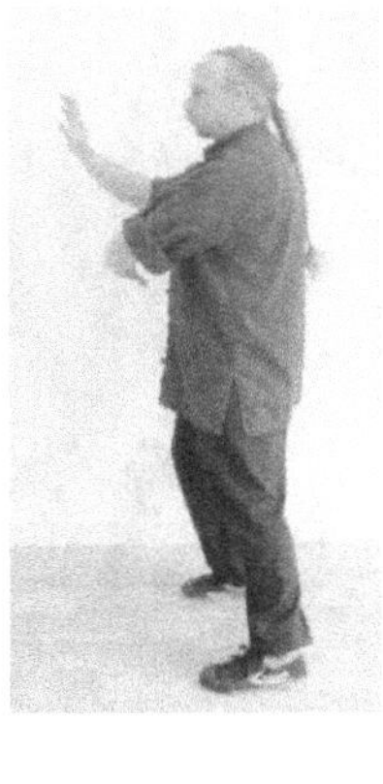

Stance: Right Leopard
Facing: South

Stance movement:
Shift the weight slightly forwards further onto the left foot and then step the right foot around and back to come into line with the left foot, pointing the toes to the front. The weight then transfers onto the right foot before correcting the left foot into the Leopard stance facing South.

Posture movement:
The right hand moves over the top of the left hand, turning it to bring the palm to facing forwards as you do so (leading with the little finger edge). As you turn to face South the right hand moves across to in front of the right shoulder (little finger edge leading) and the left hand turns to palm downwards and comes under the right elbow to finish at waist height on the right side of the body.

Move 74.

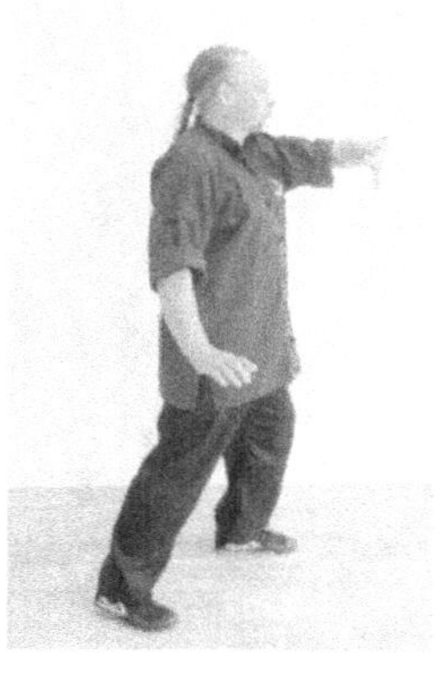 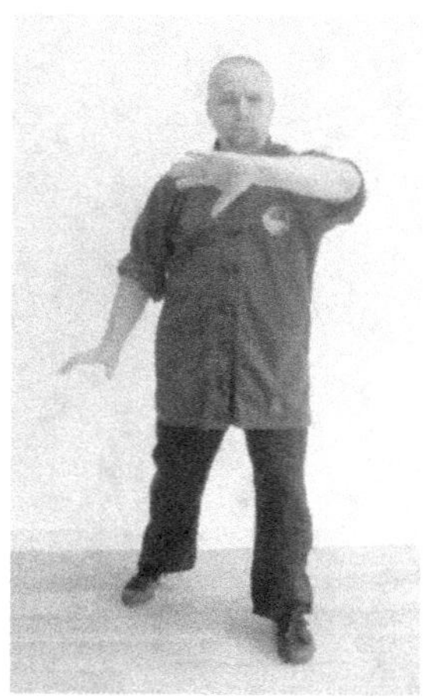

Stance: Left Dragon
Facing: South

<u>Stance movement:</u>

Step the left foot forwards and then bring the weight forwards into Dragon stance, correcting the right foot as you settle into the stance.

<u>Posture movement:</u>

The waist turns slightly to the right and then, as you move forwards, the chest opens to bring the left arm up to shoulder height with the forearm extended to the front (so think 'elbow' then 'shoulder'). The right hand presses down to finish beside the right hip.

Move 75.

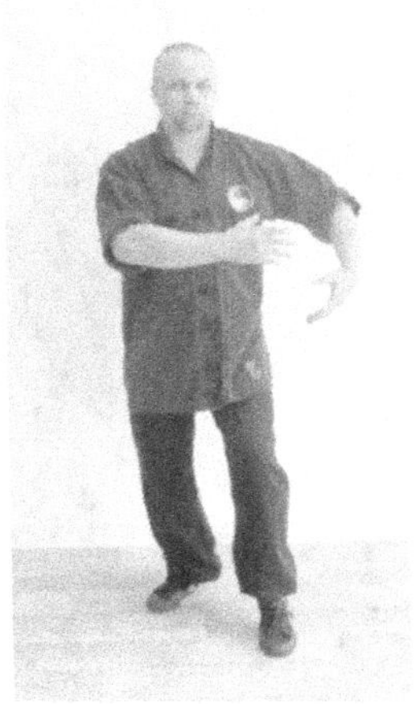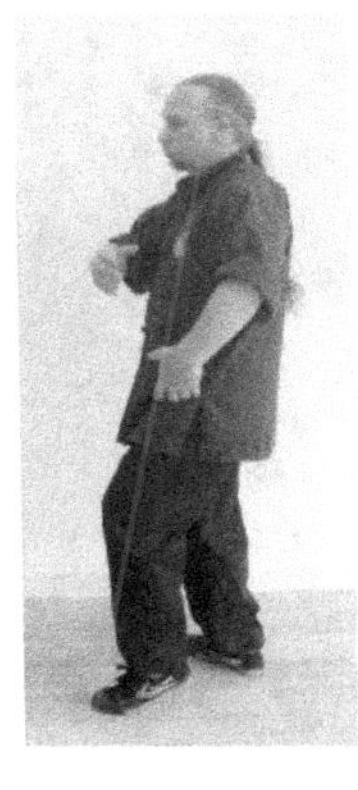

Stance: Left Cat
Facing: South

<u>Stance movement:</u>

Bring your weight back onto the right foot and draw the left foot back into a Cat stance.

<u>Posture movement:</u>

The left arm extends forwards and out to the left side (with the palm facing behind you) before rolling downwards and back in towards the body with the palm in towards the side of the body. The left arm finishes with the elbow just below shoulder height and the lower arm hanging from the elbow with the wrist slightly extended to bring the palm upwards a little with the thumb edge forwards. The right hand circles in and across the body to finish with the palm facing into the space between the left forearm and the body.

Move 76.

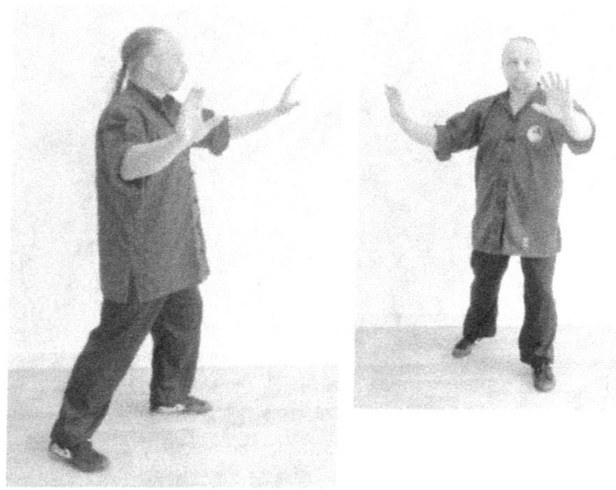

Stance: Left Dragon
Facing: East

<u>Stance movement:</u>

Step the left foot around to your left, placing the foot so that the toes are pointing to the East. Shift the weight onto the left foot and correct the right foot as you settle into the Dragon stance.

<u>Posture movement:</u>

Both hands come inwards and upwards in front of the chest (turning the upper body to the left) with the palms facing the body (still in Cat stance). Expand the chest to bring the palms to face each other as you step the left foot and then as you move into the Dragon stance both hands press outwards at shoulder height with the upper body turned approximately forty-five degrees to the right (maintaining the straight hip alignment in the Dragon stance). This brings you into position with the left hand pressing forwards and the right hand pressing out to the right.

Move 77.

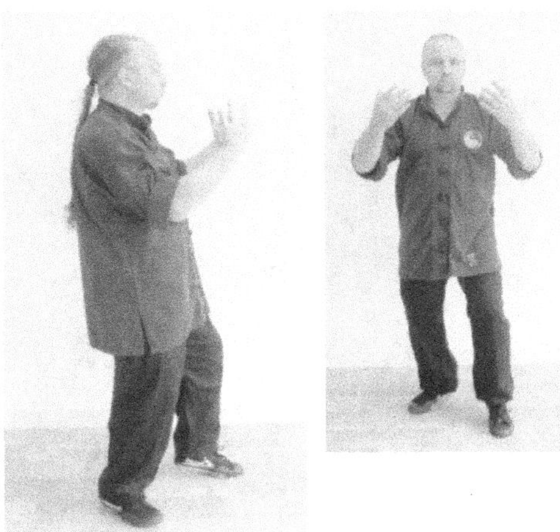

Stance: Left Cat
Facing: East

<u>Stance movement:</u>

Bring the weight back onto the right leg before drawing the left foot back into Cat stance.

<u>Posture movement:</u>

The hands continue the outwards pressing movement to roll downwards and back in. Straighten the waist as the hands continue to circle up to in front of the shoulders with the palms facing inwards (similar to the first part of movement number eight).

Move 78.

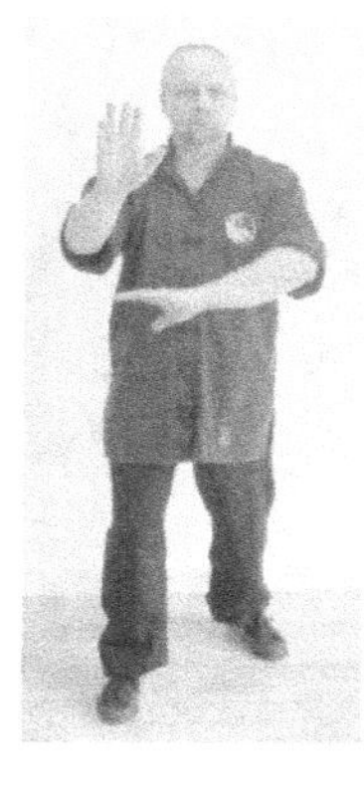 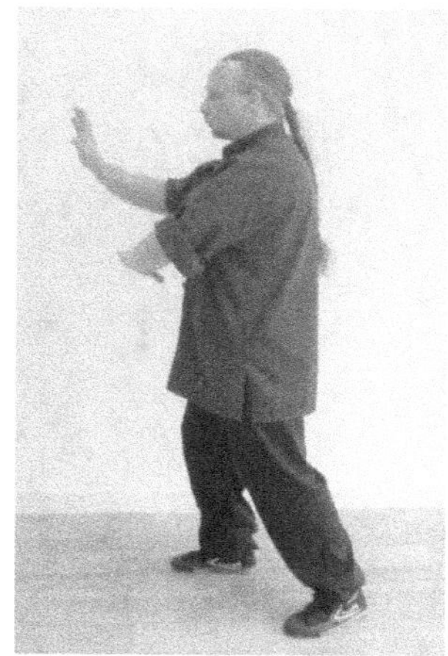

Stance: Right Dragon
Facing: West

<u>Stance movement:</u>

Place the left heel down and hook the left foot in and around to point the toes towards the South-West. Shift the weight onto the left foot, turning to your right as you do so, before stepping the right foot around and bringing the weight forward onto it in a Dragon stance facing West.

<u>Posture movement:</u>

Turn the right hand so that the palm is facing away from the body (leading with the little finger edge) and extend the hand to in front of the shoulder as you turn into Dragon. The left hand circles down and across the body to finish with the palm facing downwards at waist height on the right side of the body.

Move 79.

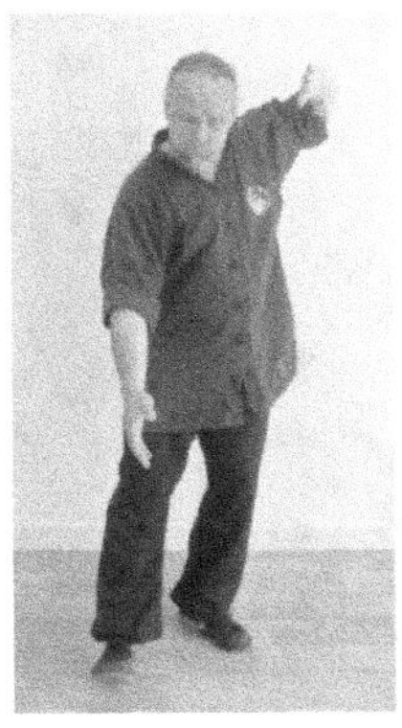 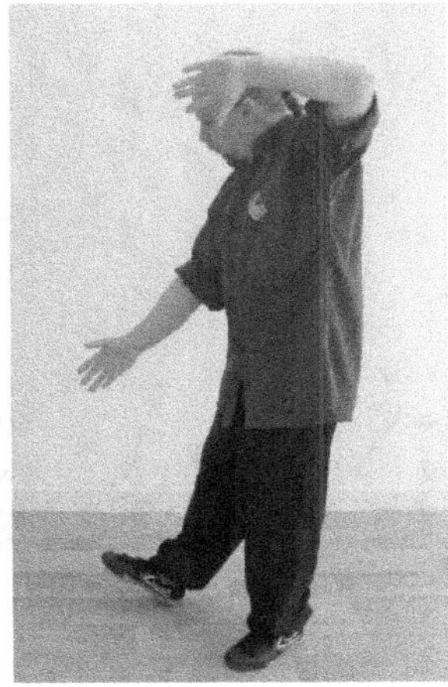

Stance: Right Monkey
Facing: West

<u>Stance movement:</u>

Draw the weight bock onto the left foot and then lift the front toes into Monkey stance.

<u>Posture movement:</u>

Extend the fingers of the right hand forwards to face the palm of the hand upwards, then roll the right hand to the right and back over to the right to bring the palm downwards. The thumb edge of the right hand then rolls upwards before the right hand 'cuts' down with the little finger edge. As the right hand cuts downwards, draw the weight back onto the left foot and lean forwards slightly from the waist. Extend the left elbow up and to the side of the head as the body turns slightly to your left (as the weight shifts) so that the left hand ends to the side of the face with the palm facing away to the left and the thumb edge downwards.

Move 80.

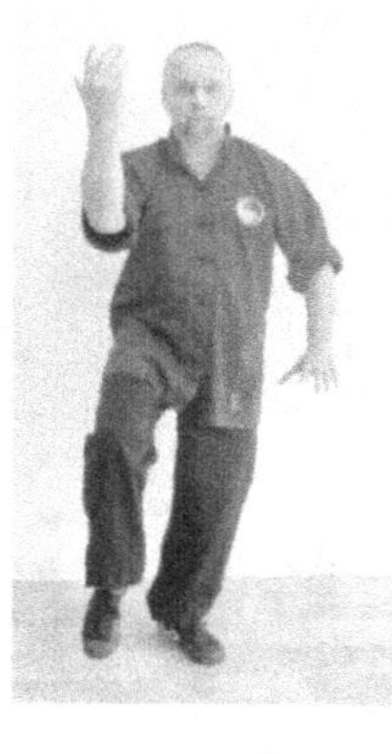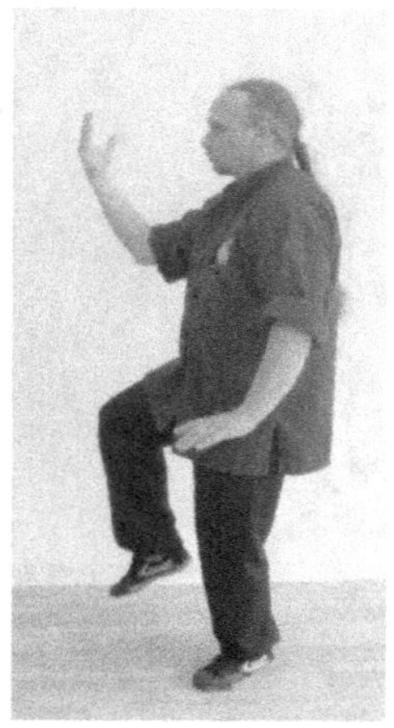

Stance: Right Crane
Facing: West

<u>Stance movement:</u>

The right leg lifts off the floor and comes up into a Crane stance in a circular movement, coming to the left as it starts to lift and then continuing outwards to the right as it comes into position for the Crane stance.

<u>Posture movement:</u>

The right arm circles inwards to the left and then outwards to the right (in an outward arm ward-off), in a similar movement to the right leg. The left arm presses down to finish palm down beside the left hip.

Move 81.

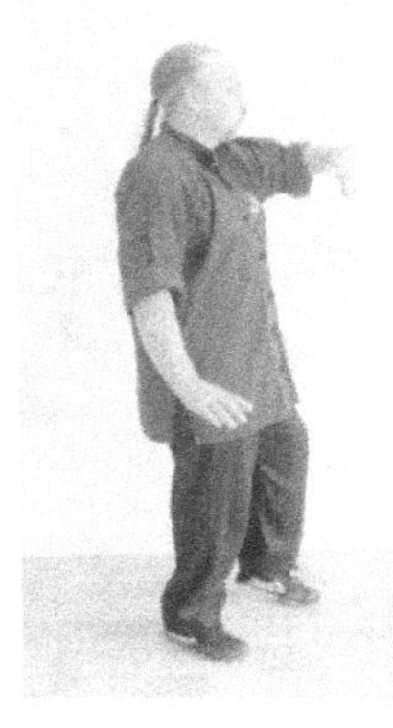 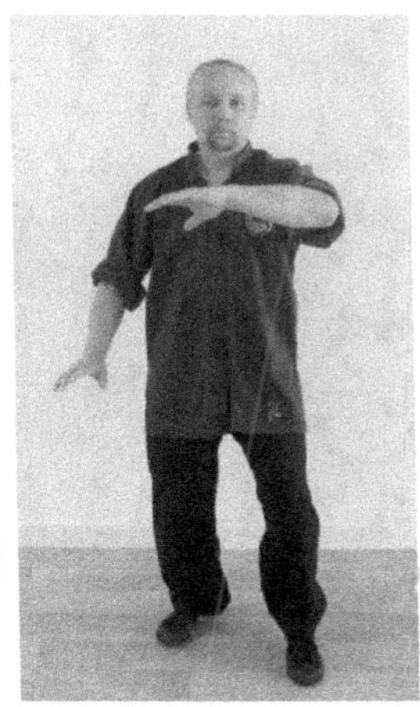

Stance: Left Cat
Facing: South

<u>Stance movement:</u>

The right foot continues the circle outward and then down and inwards until you place it back onto the floor (in the same place that it was in the Monkey stance in move Seventy-Nine). Place the heel down, correct the foot to point the toes towards the South-West and then bring the weight onto the right foot, turning the body to face South as you do so. Then draw the left foot into position for Cat stance.

<u>Posture movement:</u>

The right hand also continues its circle out and then down (with the palm facing downwards as you press down) to finish beside the right hip. The left hand comes up to chest height and then, as the body settles onto the right foot and straightens, it circles in towards the body to finish in front of the right shoulder with the palm facing downwards.

Move 82.

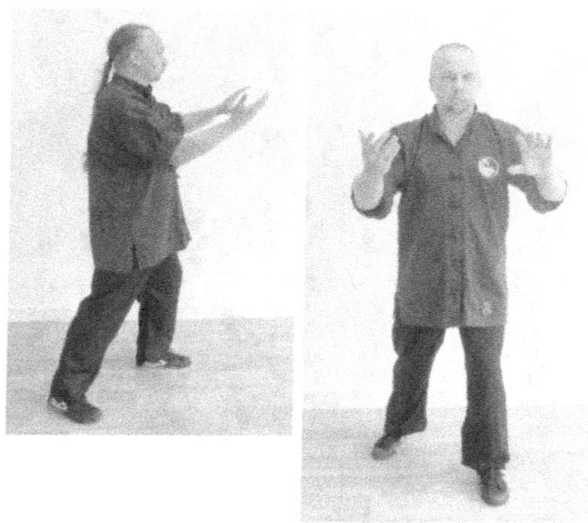

Stance: Left Dragon
Facing: South

<u>Stance movement:</u>

Step the left foot forwards and then bring the weight forwards into Dragon stance.

<u>Posture movement:</u>

The right hand comes up and across the front of the body to underneath the left elbow. Then, as you shift the weight forwards, open the chest to extend the left hand to the front (palm down at shoulder height). The right hand follows the line of the left forearm as it opens outwards (still underneath the left arm) until it opens out to the front at shoulder height with the palm facing upwards.

Move 83.

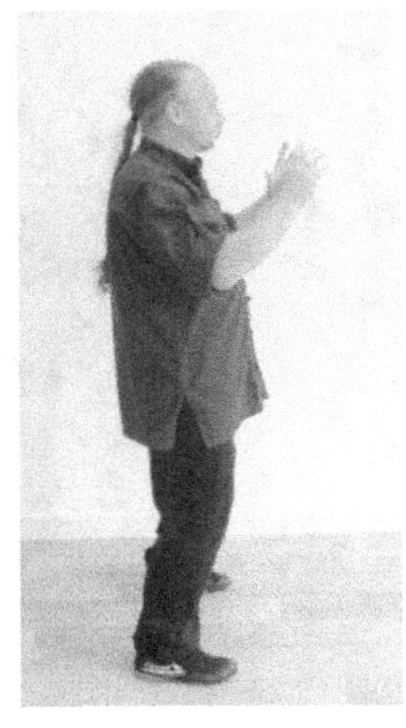 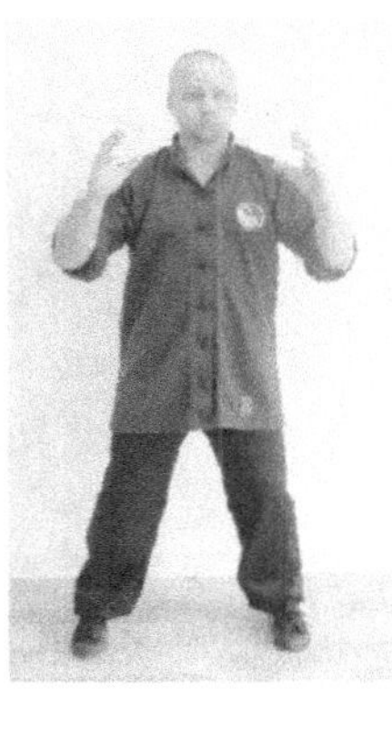

Stance: Riding Horse
Facing: East

Stance movement:

Sink the weight back onto the right foot and then step the left foot behind you, placing it in line with the right foot with the toes pointing to the East. Bring the weight onto the left foot, turning to the East as you do so, and then correct the right foot before settling the weight into Riding Horse stance.

Posture movement:

The right hand opens slightly to the right and then turn both hands to face each other as you start to shift the weight backwards. As the body turns and settles into Riding Horse, hold a 'ball' with the hands in front of the shoulders and the fingers pointing upwards.

Move 84.

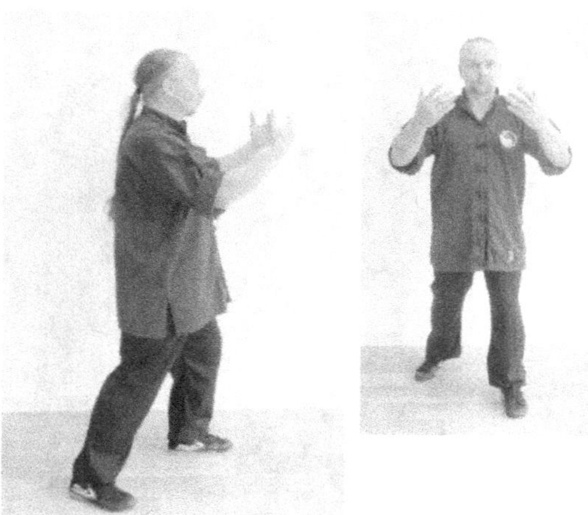

Stance: Left Dragon
Facing: East

<u>Stance movement:</u>

Draw the weight onto the right foot and then step the left foot forwards to come into Dragon stance.

<u>Posture movement:</u>

The hands press down (with the fingers pointing towards each other and palms down) to upper abdomen height. They then turn in towards the body and come up to in front of the shoulders (with palms facing the body – two 'semi-circles' similar to start of movement number eight). Then 'press' forwards with the back of the hands (again, similar to movement number eight).

<u>Timing:</u>

Time the hands pressing downwards and rising up to shoulder height to coincide with the shift of the weight onto the right foot.

Move 85.

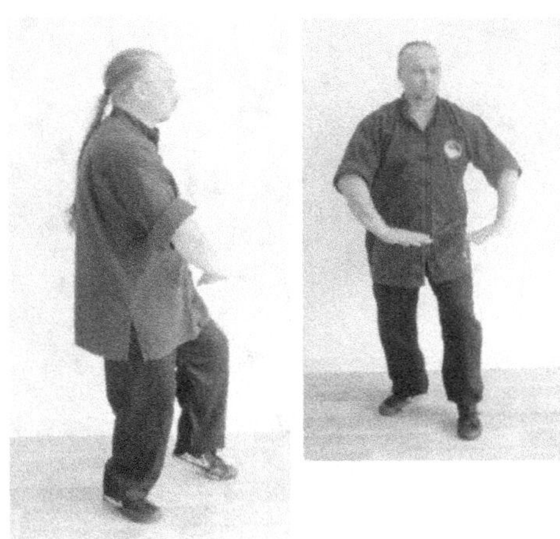

Stance: Left Cat
Facing: East

<u>Stance movement:</u>

Shift the weight back onto the right foot and then draw the left foot up into Cat stance.

<u>Posture movement:</u>

As your weight moves back onto the right foot allow the hands to come down to waist height with palms upwards (fingers pointing forwards). Then, roll the hands up and to the sides to bring them to palms down in front of the shoulders with fingertips pointing towards fingertips. Press the hands downwards to Lower Tantien height (with the waist turned slightly to the left to bring the hands to either side of the knee) as you sink the weight into the Cat stance.

Move 86.

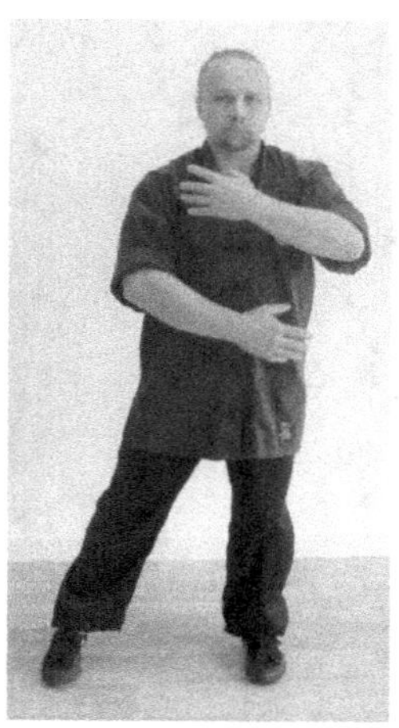

Stance: Left Leopard
Facing: South

<u>Stance movement:</u>

Step the left foot forwards and to your right, before shifting the weight onto it and correcting the right foot to come into Leopard stance facing South.

<u>Posture movement:</u>

Both hands continue to press down and outwards. They then continue their circles to come back inwards toward the front of the body (as if 'embracing' yourself). Finishing with the left hand's palm facing the right shoulder and the right hand palm facing the body at waist height on the left side of the body.

Move 87.

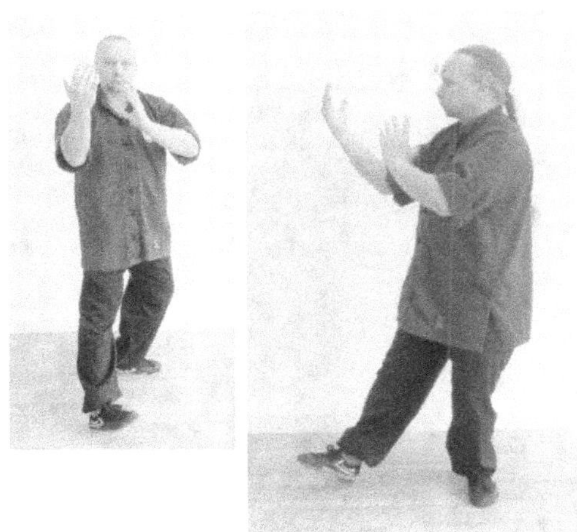

Stance: Right Monkey
Facing: West

<u>Stance movement:</u>

Turn the hips towards the South-West and raise the toes of the right foot to come into a Monkey stance (with the stance on an angle towards the South-West).

<u>Posture movement:</u>

The upper body turns all the way to the right to face West (so there is a twist of the waist with the shoulders facing West and the hips facing South-West). The right hand opens up and outwards to slightly higher than shoulder height with the palm facing inwards towards the body (in an outward arm ward-off). The left hand drifts across to its position in front of the chest.

Move 88.

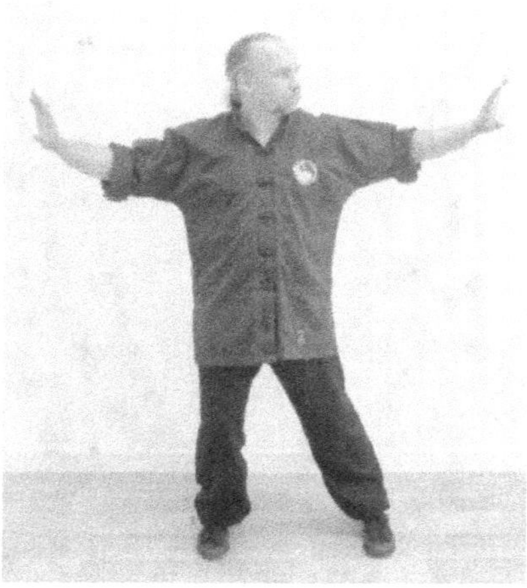

Stance: Right Leopard
Facing: South

<u>Stance movement:</u>

Replace the right foot onto the ground with the toes pointing to the South and then bring your weight across into the Right Leopard stance.

<u>Posture movement:</u>

The arms come down in front of the body to waist height and then continue their circles up and to the sides to finish at shoulder height with the palms facing away from the body. The head turns to look at the back of the left hand.

Move 89.

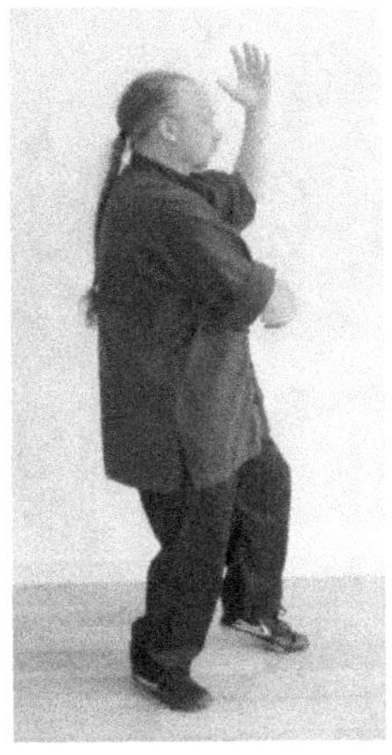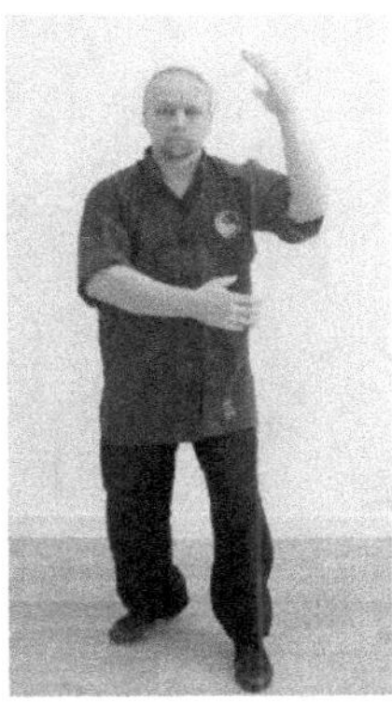

Stance: Left Cat
Facing: East

<u>Stance movement:</u>

Move the weight over onto the left leg and correct the right foot to point towards the South-East. Shift the weight back onto the right foot, turning the body to face East and then draw the left foot into Cat stance.

<u>Posture movement:</u>

The left arm moves up into an outward arm ward-off position defending the head and the right arm 'wraps' around the waist, drawing the left foot in as it comes inwards.

Move 90.

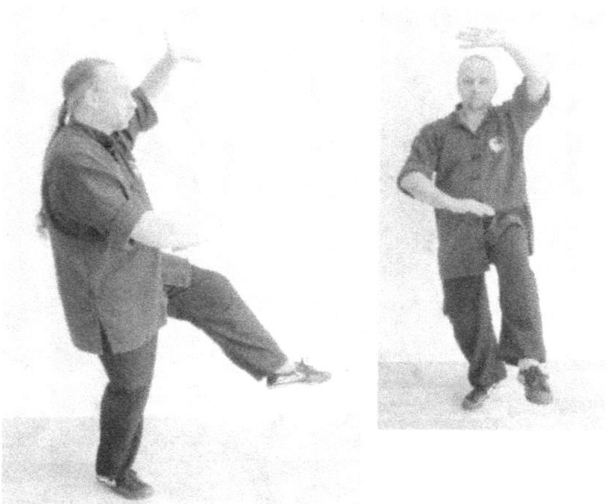

Stance: Left Dog
Facing: East

Stance movement:

The left leg lifts into Dog stance, remembering to drop the toes into the stance (so stepping 'heel-toe' on the air).

Posture movement:

The right hand rolls across the waist (palm upwards) and then circles up on the right side of the body to chest height. It then continues its circle to face palm down in front of the chest before pressing downwards along the centre-line. The left elbow raises, bringing the left hand up into a 'salute' position. You should have a feeling of pressing both palms outwards away from the centre at the end of the movement.

Timing:

The movement of the left arm should last the full duration of the movement. The right hand raises as the leg lifts, before pressing down as you settle into the stance (heel-toe).

Move 91.

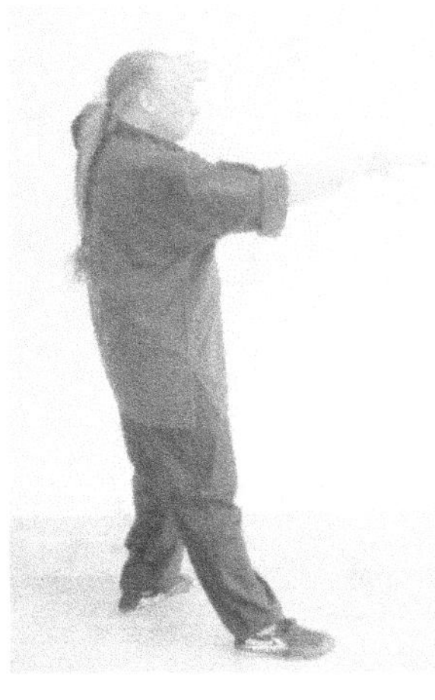 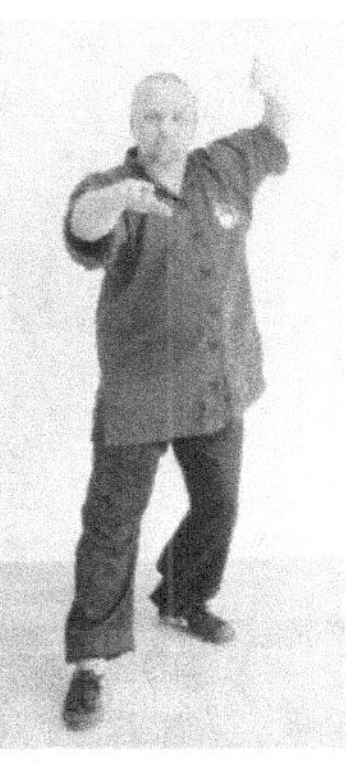

Stance: Right Duck
Facing: East

<u>Stance movement:</u>

The left leg swings down and to the left to land behind the body. The weight is then shifted back onto the left foot into Right Duck stance.

<u>Posture movement:</u>

The body turns towards the left slightly, bringing the left hand to the side of the head. The right hand circles to the left and then extends outwards to point forwards with the palm down at shoulder height (opening the chest).

Move 92.

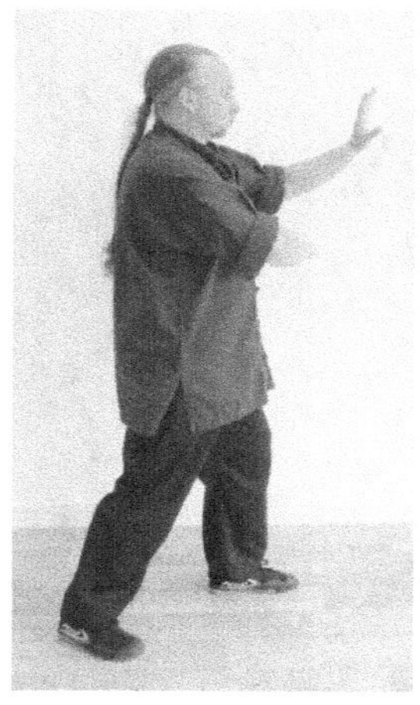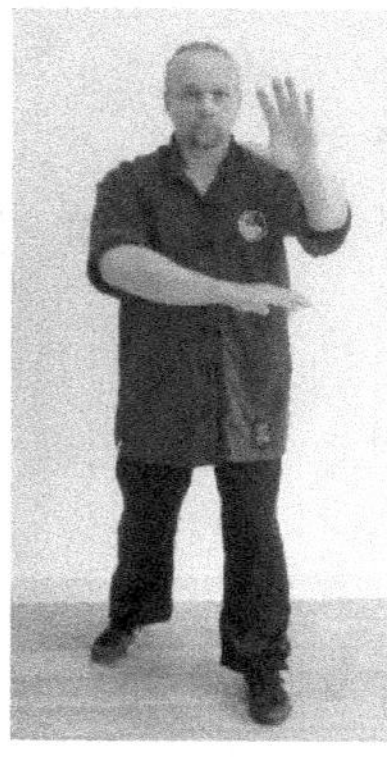

Stance: Left Dragon
Facing: East

<u>Stance movement:</u>

Step the left foot forwards and then shift the weight forwards onto it into a Dragon stance.

<u>Posture movement:</u>

Expand the chest further so that the right hand continues its circle from the previous movement (outwards to the right and then inwards across the body) so that it finishes palm downwards at waist height on the left side of the body. As you come forward into the Dragon stance, straighten the body and bring the left hand forwards at shoulder height with the palm facing forwards away from the body.

Move 93.

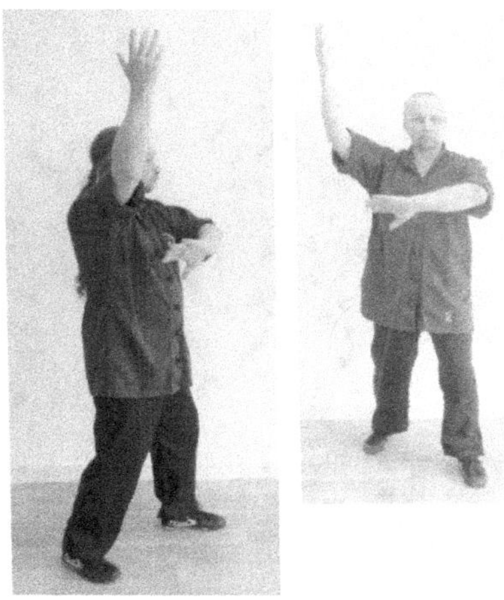

Stance: Left Snake
Facing: East

<u>Stance movement:</u>

Draw the weight back onto the right leg (into Duck stance) before shifting forwards again into Snake stance (being careful not to go too far and end in Dragon).

<u>Posture movement:</u>

Both arms circle downwards and towards the right side of the body. Turn the body to the right as the arms continue their circle before straightening the body as the right arm moves to the top of its arc (finishing pointing upwards from the shoulder) and the left arm rolls to in front of the body with the forearm extended. The left hand finishes at chest height in front of the right side of the body with the palm at a forty-five degree angle (much like movement number Thirty One).

Move 94.

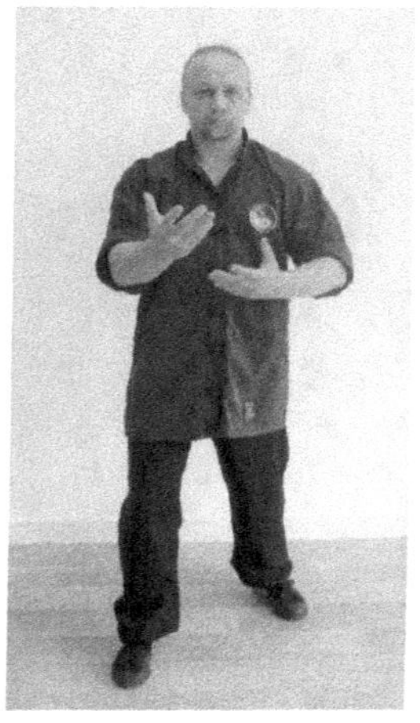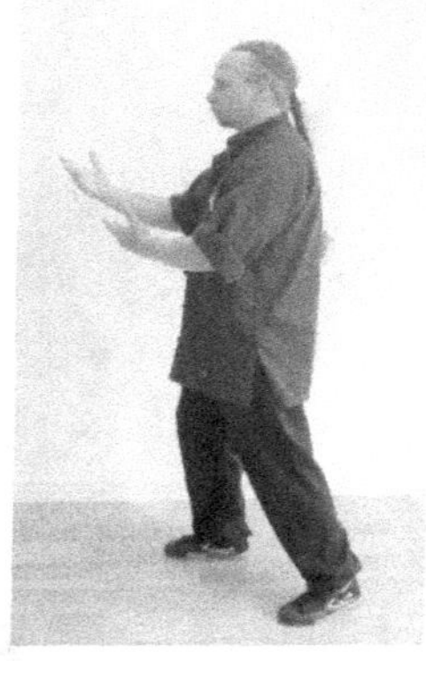

Stance: Right Dragon
Facing: South

<u>Stance movement:</u>

Draw the weight back onto the right foot and then correct the left foot so that the toes are pointing towards the South-East. Step the right foot towards the South pointing the toes forwards and then bring the weight forwards into the Dragon stance facing South.

<u>Posture movement:</u>

Expand the chest to roll the shoulders outwards, 'reversing' the directions of each arm's circle. The arms then circle down and to the sides before coming to in front of the body with the palms facing upwards. The hands 'scoop' forwards and upwards to finish with the left fingertips pointing towards the right wrist (similar to movement number Four)

<u>Timing:</u>

The arms circle down towards the waist as you shift the weight back and correct the left foot, they then come forwards as you step the right foot and shift into Dragon stance.

Move 95.

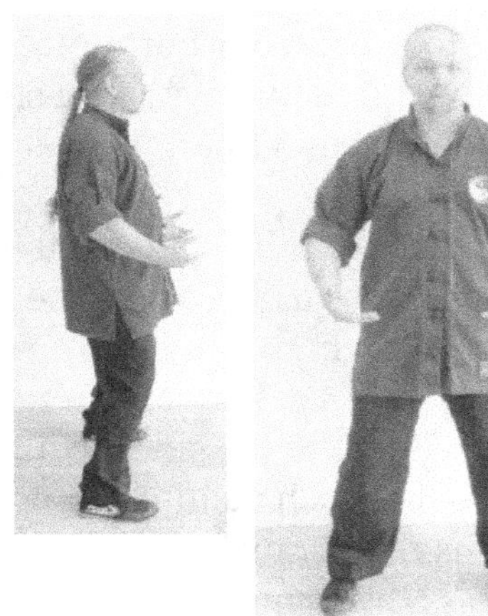

Stance: Riding Horse
Facing: South

<u>Stance movement:</u>

Draw the weight back onto the left foot, then step the right foot back to in line with the left foot, pointing the toes to face forwards. Shift the weight slightly onto the right foot in order to correct the left foot before settling into Riding Horse stance.

<u>Posture movement:</u>

The arms continue their forward and upward movement to chest height before opening out to the sides and turning the hands palms down. Continue to circle the hands back towards the sides of the body before turning the palms upwards as the hands come to just in front of the hips at Tantien height. At the end of the movement the fingertips should be pointing slightly forwards as the elbows settle into position.

Gather Earth's Energy.

If you are choosing to finish your Form practice at this point (the end of Movement Number Ninety-Five), you should then perform the sequence 'Gather Earth's Energy' as detailed at the end of the Short Form in Book One.

To initiate the sequence from the end of Movement Ninety-Five, lower the hands to your sides as you draw the left foot into Eagle Stance, then continue the arm movements up and to the sides to shoulder height.

The arms then return down to the sides, before coming up in front of the body to cross so that each palm is facing the front of the opposite shoulder. The arms then draw back down in front of the body, uncrossing as they pass the Tantien to finish by the sides.

Section 3.

Taiji Feishou Form.

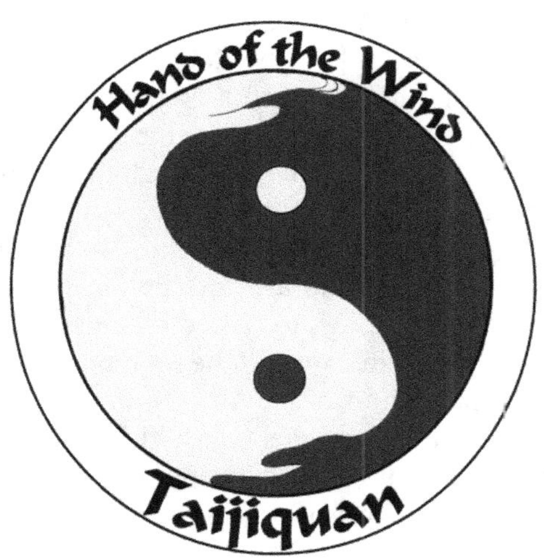

Taiji Feishou Form

In Book One, To the Ede of the Cyclone, the movements of the Feishou Form were described up to movement number thirty. The next section continues on from this point and describes movements from thirty-one to movement number sixty.

The Feishou Form follows the same principles as the Tai Chi Form and should therefore be considered to have the same level of detail within it. There are differences between the two Forms – most notably that the Feishou is directed more from the Middle Tantien than the Tai Chi Form (particularly the Short Form) and it is this that gives the Feishou its more expansive feel. Do not allow it to lose the grounded-ness though – be very aware of powering the movements through the Bubbling Spring points and ensure that your stances are effective.

There is a huge amount of learning to be found within the Feishou Form for those students who are prepared to put the time and effort into refining the movements. All too often it is just seen as 'just another Form to learn' and students rarely spend the required time practicing the Feishou to gain a real appreciation of it. As with the Tai Chi Form, every posture and every transitional movement should be examined and performed in accordance with all of the Tai Chi principles and gaining an understanding of the martial applications of the movements will advance your Tai Chi skill level immeasurably.

Feishou Form Quick Reference Table

Move	Stance	Facing
30	Right Cat	East
31	Left Duck	East
32	Right Duck	East
33	Left Duck	East
34	Left Duck	East
35	Right Cat	East
36	Left Cat	East
37	Left Crane	East
38	Left Dog	East
39	Right Chicken	East
40	Left Dragon	East
41	Right Dragon	West
42	Right Dragon	West
43	Left Dragon	East
44	Left Crane	East
45	Left Dragon	East
46	Left Leopard	South
47	Right Dragon	West
48	Left Dragon	West
49	Left Leopard	North
50	Right Dragon	East
51	Right Dragon	East
52	Left Dragon	East
53	Left Leopard	South
54	Right Dragon	West
55	Left Dragon	East
56	Left Crane	East
57	Left Dragon	East
58	Eagle	South
59	Eagle	South
60	Left Dragon	East

Move 30.

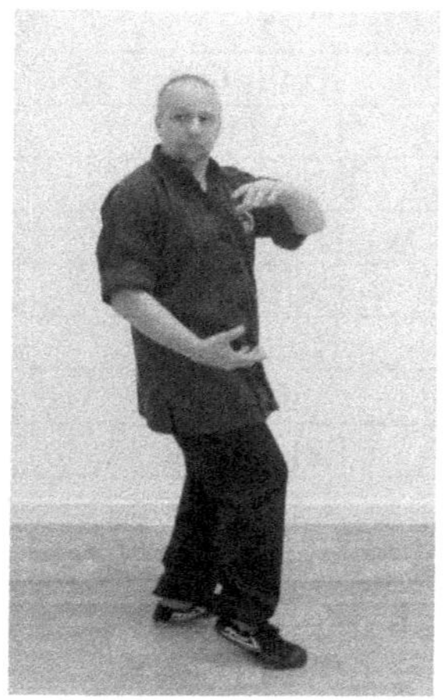

Stance: Right Cat
Facing: East

This is the position arrived at in the last of the movements of the Feishou Form as described in Book One: To the Edge of the Cyclone.

The movement is therefore not described here but the image is presented as a reminder.

The following pages will describe the movements of the Feishou Form from number Thirty-One to number Sixty.

Move 31.

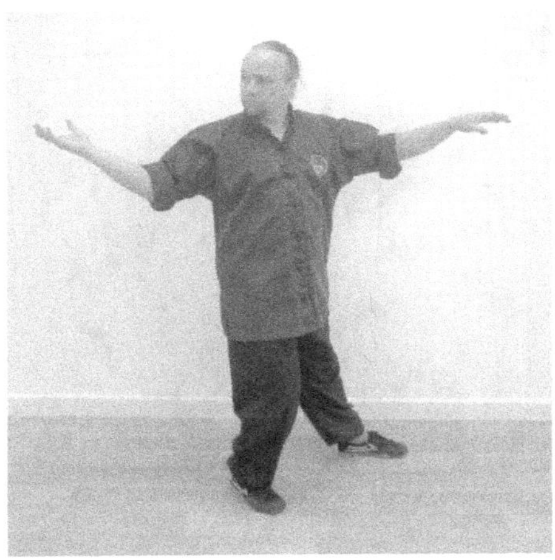

Stance: Left Duck
Facing: East

Stance movement:

Step the right foot back behind you and shift the weight back onto it to come into a Left Duck stance.

Posture movement:

The arms separate outwards as the upper body turns to the right to finish with both arms at shoulder height (right hand palm upwards and left hand palm downwards). The hips should still be facing towards the East with the upper body turned to the right from the waist – this results in the left arm pointing Eastwards and the right arm pointing behind you towards the West. The head should also turn to the right so that you end up looking at the right hand behind you.

Move 32.

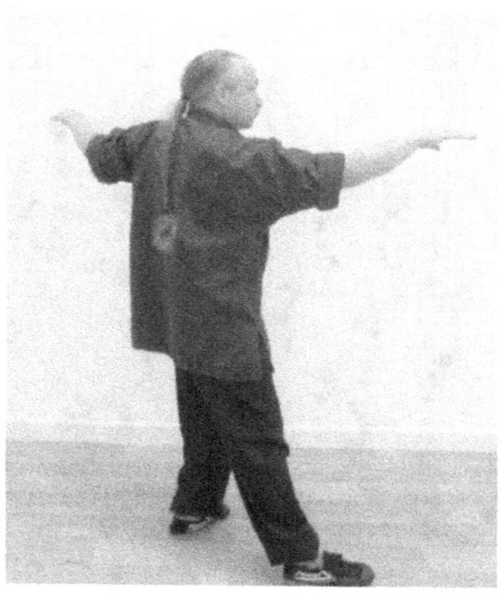

Stance: Right Duck
Facing: East

<u>Stance movement:</u>

Step the left foot behind you before shifting the weight onto it to come into a Right Duck stance.

<u>Posture movement:</u>

The arms drift down towards waist height as you step the left foot, then they drift back up to shoulder height with both palms facing downwards. Again, the upper body is turned so that the right arm is pointing forwards and the left arm is pointing backwards although this time the head is looking forwards.

Move 33.

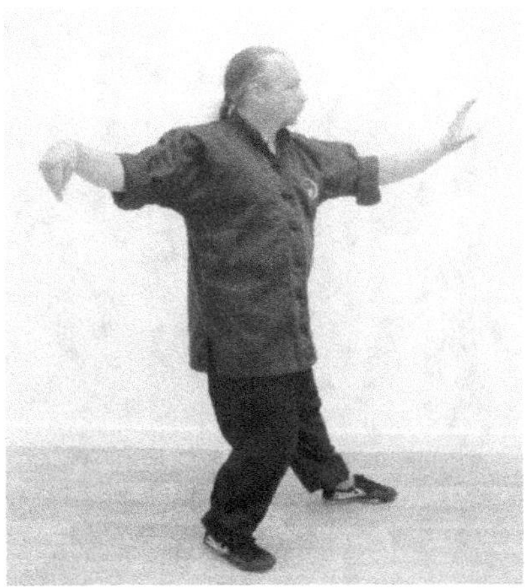

Stance: Left Duck
Facing: East

<u>Stance movement:</u>

Once again, step the right foot back to behind you and transfer the weight back into the Left Duck stance.

<u>Posture movement:</u>

As in the previous movement, the arms drift down and then up and the body turns to the right. The head remains looking forwards and the left hand is fingers upwards with the palm facing the front. The right hand fingers are pointing downwards in a 'Crane's Head' position.

Move 34.

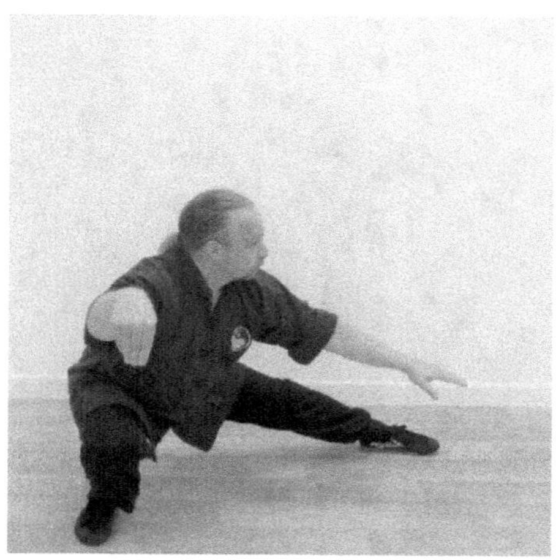

Stance: Left Duck
Facing: East

<u>Stance movement:</u>

'Push' out of the left foot to step the right foot further back behind you and then drop down into a deep Left Duck stance.

<u>Posture movement:</u>

The left hand makes a big sweeping circle to the right side of the body and downwards to finish palm downwards above the left foot. The body straightens a bit back towards the East as the right hand traces a small circle (anticlockwise) to finish at shoulder height extended to the right side of the body (still in 'Crane's Head').

<u>Notes:</u>

The depth of the Duck stance is dependant on how flexible you are – do not feel that you have to go as deep into the stance as the picture above if you are not able to! The picture to the right shows a perfectly acceptable posture for this movement!

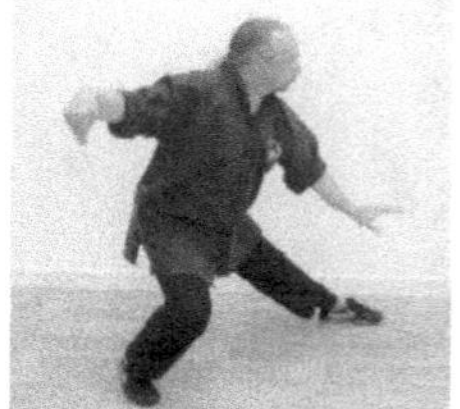

Move 35.

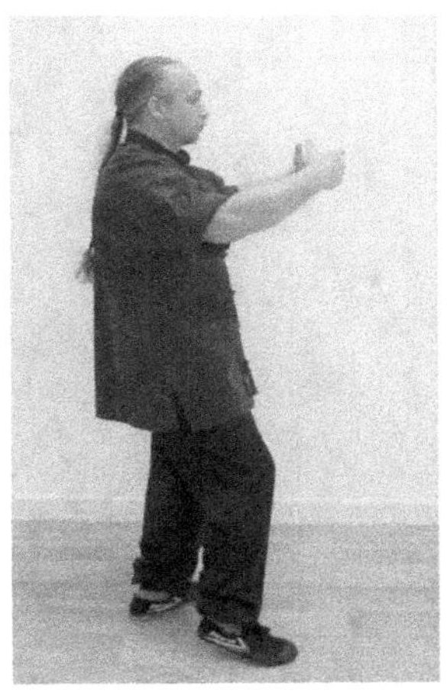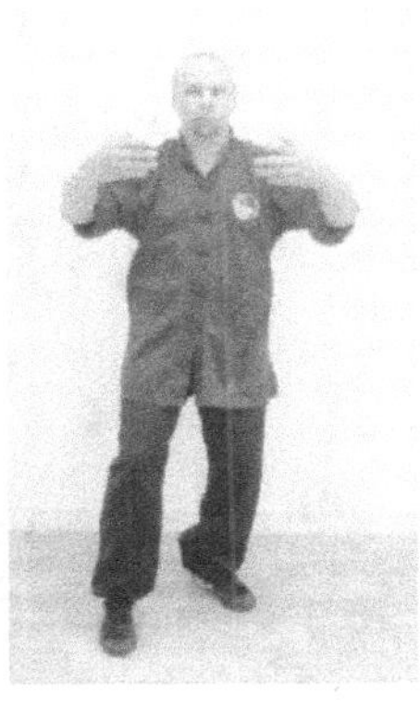

Stance: Right Cat
Facing: East

<u>Stance movement:</u>

'Bounce' back up out of the right leg, bringing the weight forwards onto the left leg and then stepping the right foot forwards to come into the Cat stance.

<u>Posture movement:</u>

The left hand continues its circle out to the left side of the body. Both hands then circle inwards at chest height to finish in front of the shoulders, palms facing inwards with the thumb edge upwards so that the tips of the fingers are pointing towards each other.

Move 36.

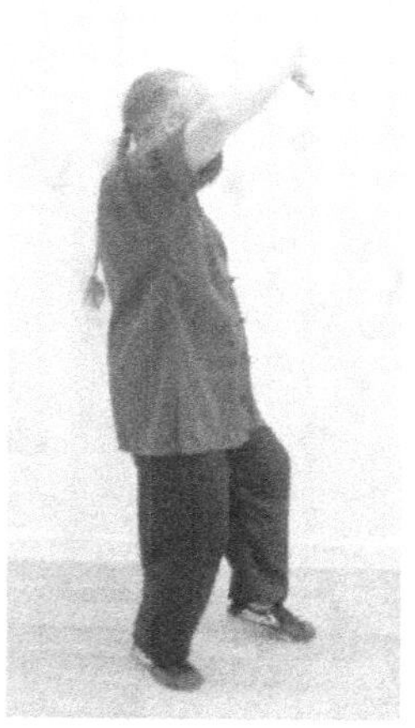 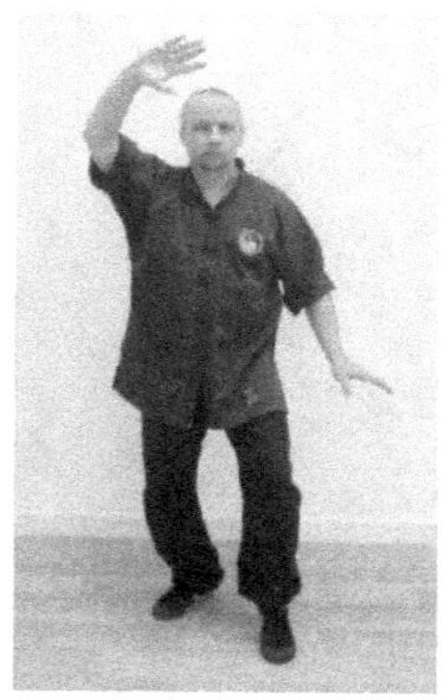

Stance: Left Cat
Facing: East

<u>Stance movement:</u>

Step the right foot directly backwards and then bring the weight back onto it, drawing the left foot into Cat stance.

<u>Posture movement:</u>

Both hands draw downwards in front of the body (with the palms still facing the body) to below waist height. The right hand then circles up and out to the right side of the body to come back into a 'salute' position. The left hand makes a small circle at approximately waist height to finish with the palm downwards beside the left hip.

Move 37.

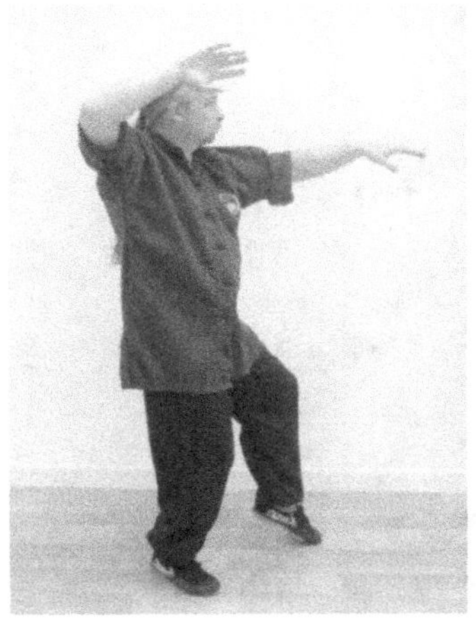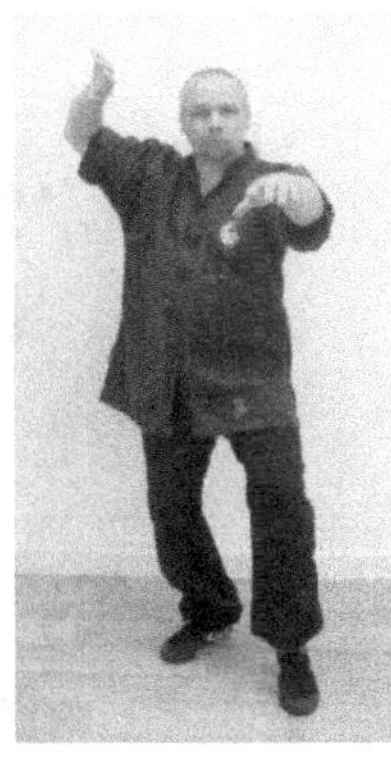

Stance: Left Cat/Crane
Facing: East

<u>Stance movement:</u>

Spin a full three hundred and sixty degrees on the right foot to come back to facing East. Ideally, you should aim to keep the toes of the right foot just off the floor in a Crane stance at the end of the spin, but many students will find it easier to allow the toes to lightly touch the floor at this point.

<u>Posture movement:</u>

The left hand comes up and outwards to shoulder height with the palm facing downwards (bringing the arm up as you initiate the 'spin' and maintaining the arm position at shoulder height throughout the 'spin'). At the end of the 'spin' the waist turns around forty-five degrees to the right which brings the left arm towards the front of the body. The right hand stays up in its 'salute' position but at the end of the movement as the waist turns to the right, the movement of the upper body brings the hand to the right side of the head.

Move 38.

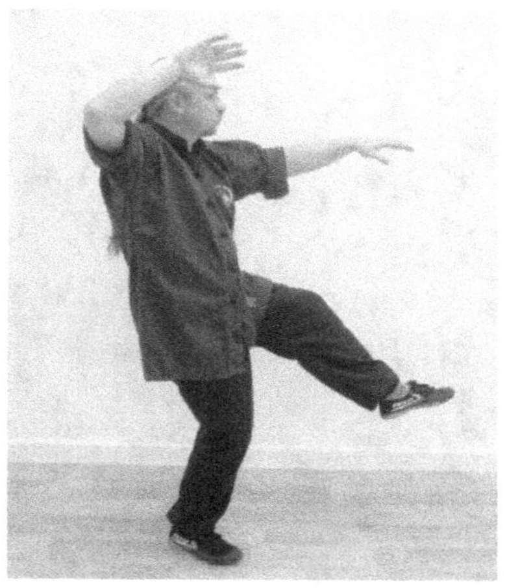

Stance: Left Dog
Facing: East

<u>Stance movement:</u>

The left leg lifts up into Dog stance.

<u>Posture movement:</u>

The arms and upper body maintain the same position from the end of the previous movement.

Move 39.

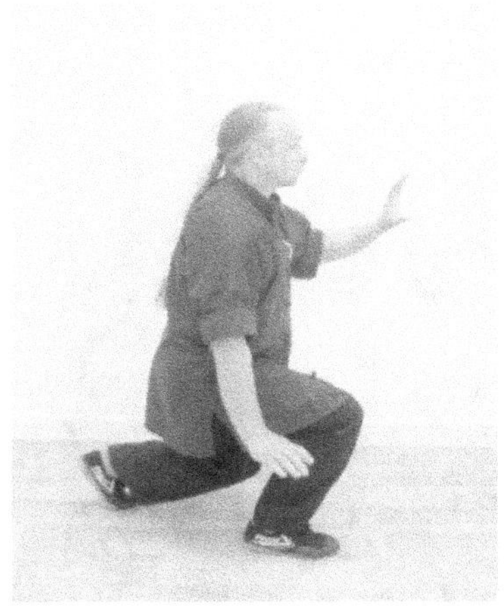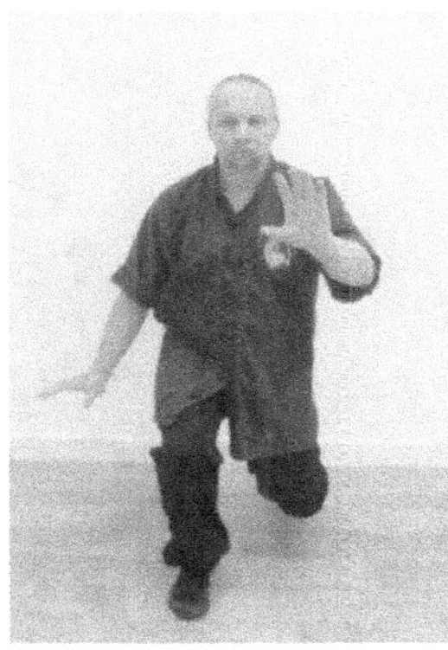

Stance: Right Chicken
Facing: East

<u>Stance movement:</u>

The left leg swings back down to place the foot behind you (with the ball of the foot on the floor and the heel lifted), lowering the weight on the right foot to come into a Chicken stance.

<u>Posture movement:</u>

The left hand 'rolls' back and towards the body to finish with the palm facing forwards in front of the left shoulder. The right hand presses downwards with the palm facing the floor until it is beside the right hip.

Move 40.

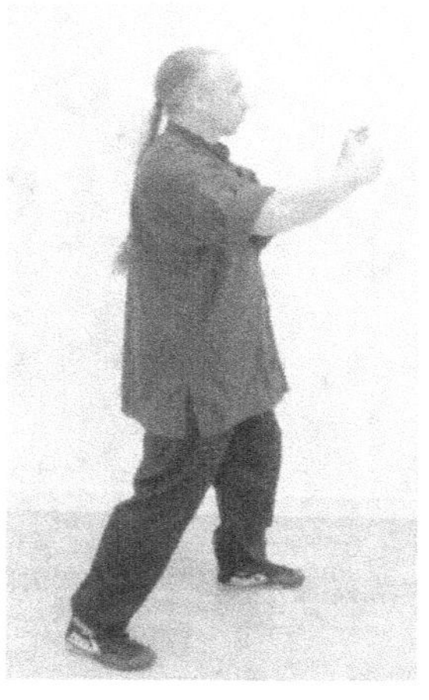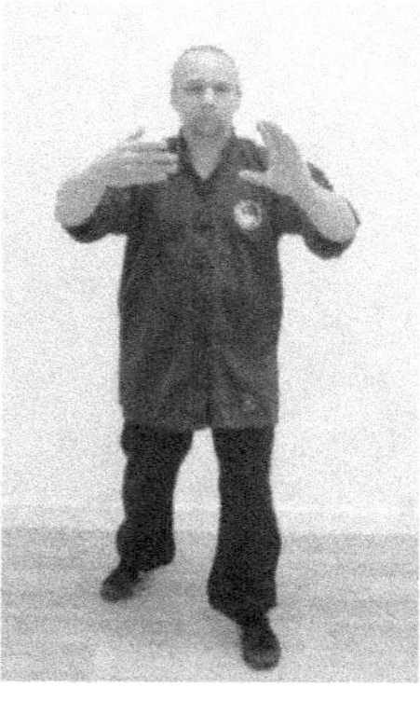

Stance: Left Dragon
Facing: East

<u>Stance movement:</u>

Step the left foot forwards, bringing the weight onto it. Correct the back foot as you settle into the Dragon stance.

<u>Posture movement:</u>

The right hand circles up and inwards to chest height (finishing in front of the right shoulder with the palm facing the chest and the thumb edge on top). The left hand extends slightly forwards, angling the little finger edge slightly ahead of the thumb edge (so that the hand is held at approximately a forty-five degree angle). The finger tips of the right hand should be pointing at the Laogong point in the middle of the left palm.

Move 41.

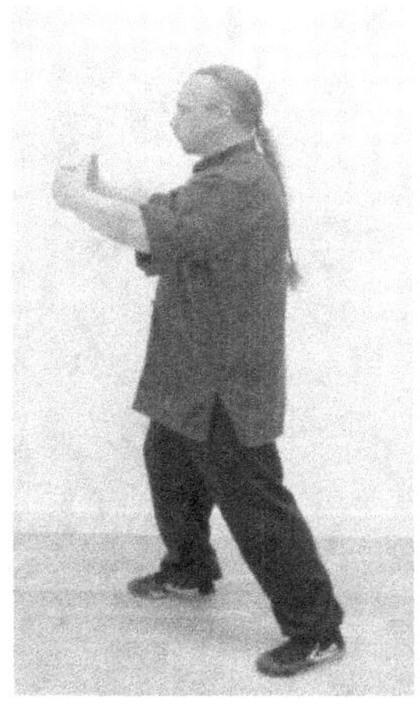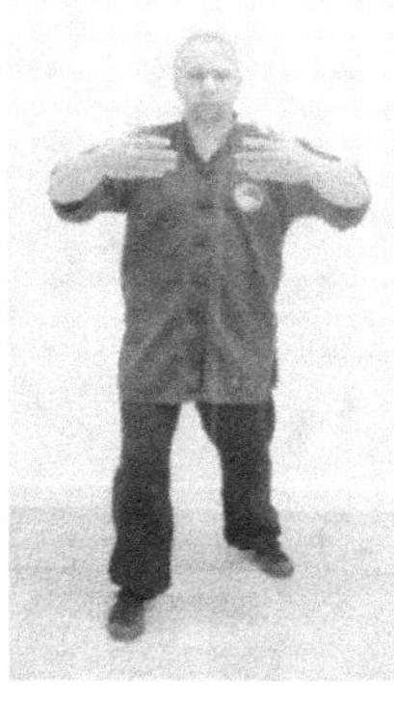

Stance: Right Dragon
Facing: West

<u>Stance movement:</u>

The weight shifts back onto the right foot, then correct the left foot (turning it to point towards the South-West). Bring the weight onto the left foot, step the right foot around to point West and then shift the weight forwards into the Dragon stance.

<u>Posture movement:</u>

As the left foot is corrected, the left hand turns so that the palm is facing the body with thumb edge upwards (fingertips of each hand facing towards each other). Maintain this hand position throughout the rest of the movement.

Move 42.

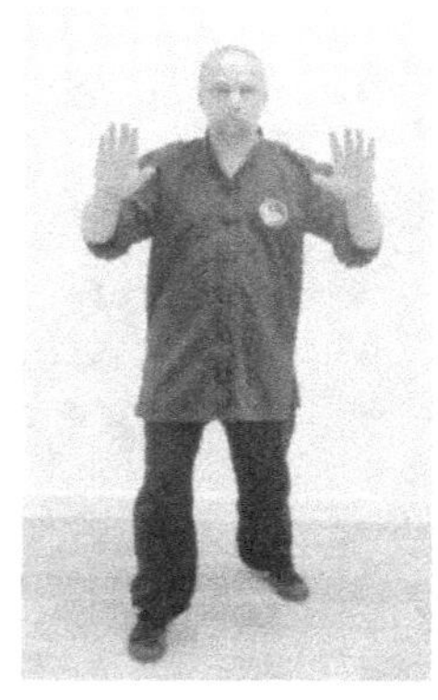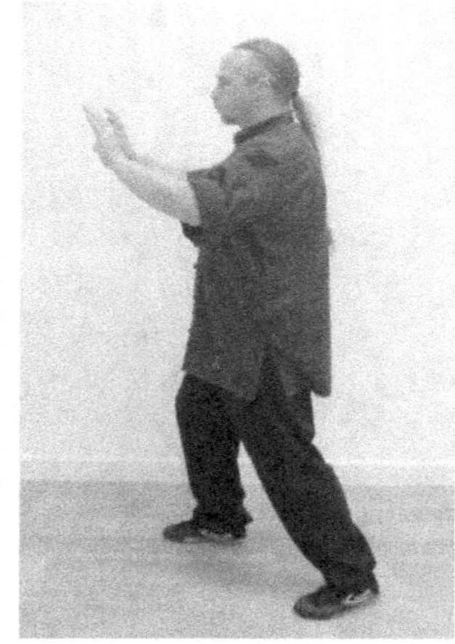

Stance: Right Dragon
Facing: West

<u>Stance movement:</u>

Maintain the same Dragon stance throughout this movement.

<u>Posture movement:</u>

The hands roll back towards the body before 'pushing' forwards with the palms.

Move 43.

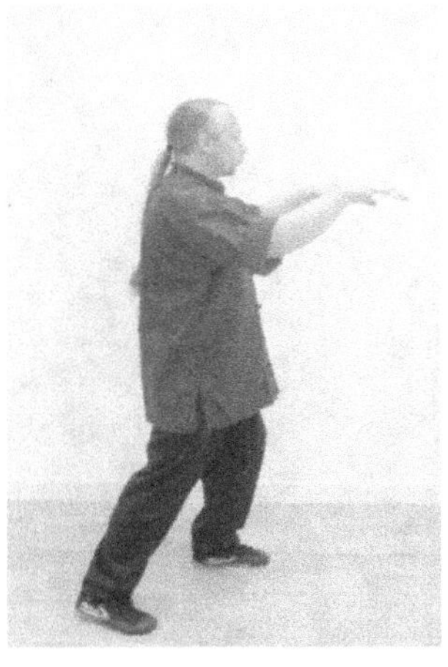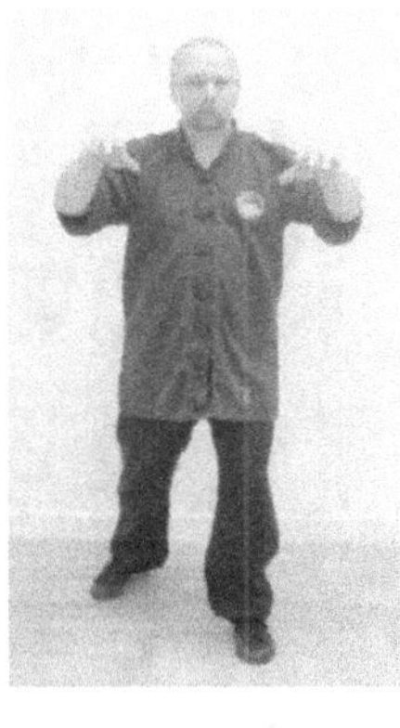

Stance: Left Dragon
Facing: East

<u>Stance movement:</u>

Draw the weight back onto the left foot and then correct the right foot to point towards the South-East. Shift your weight onto the right foot and step the left foot around to face East before moving forwards onto it to come into Dragon stance.

<u>Posture movement:</u>

The arms drift down to waist height as the weight shifts onto the left foot and the then drift back up to shoulder height as you come into the Left Dragon stance (with the palms facing downwards).

Move 44.

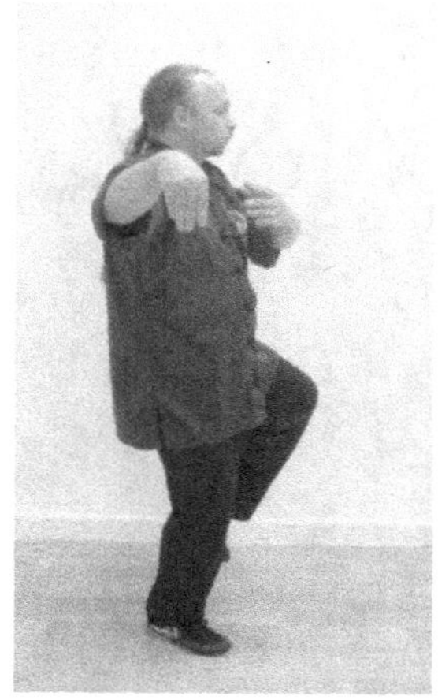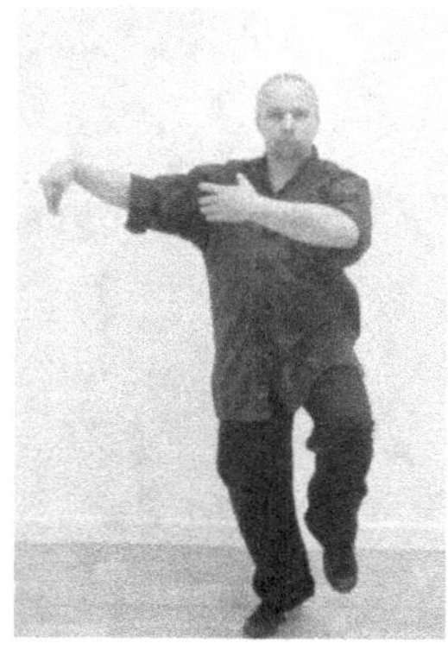

Stance: Left Crane
Facing: East

<u>Stance movement:</u>

Draw the weight back onto the right leg and lift the left le up into a Crane stance (remembering that in the Feishou, the foot is pulled back rather than just hanging down as it would be in the Tai Chi Form).

<u>Posture movement:</u>

Both hands drift down to waist height and then continue the circle to come back up to shoulder height. The right arm is extended with the hand 'hanging' downwards and the left arm is bent with the palm of the hand facing the body. Turn the waist a little so that the left hand is in front of the right shoulder and the right arm is extended out to the right side of the body.

<u>Timing:</u>

The hands drift down as the weight shifts backwards and then rise as you lift the leg into Crane.

Move 45.

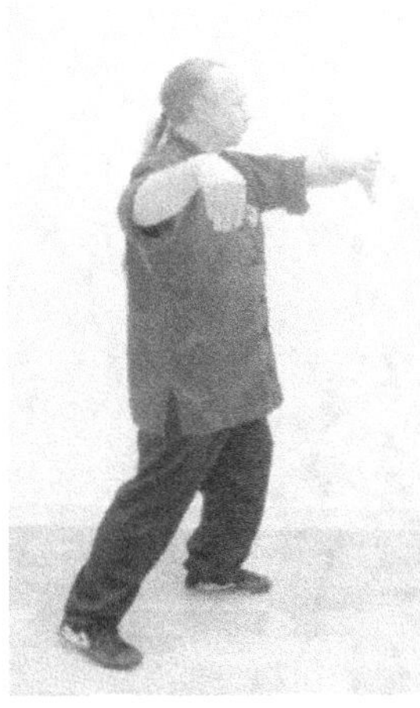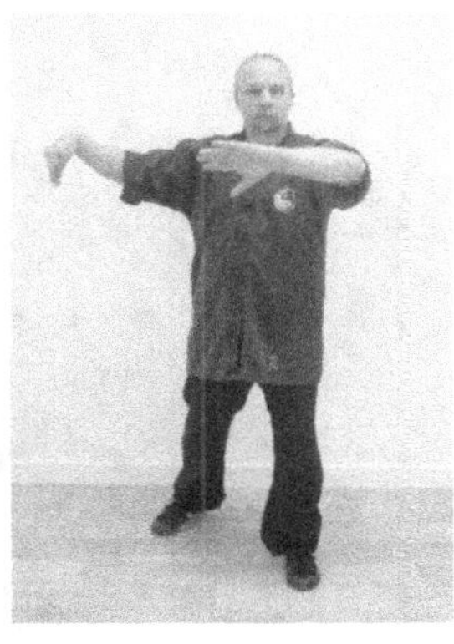

Stance: Left Dragon
Facing: East

<u>Stance movement:</u>

Step the left foot down in front of the body and bring the weight forwards onto it into the Dragon stance.

<u>Posture movement:</u>

The left hand follows a circle down and forwards before 'scooping' back up to chest height. The right hand makes a small circle (anti-clockwise) at shoulder height – ensure the timing is such that both hands finish their movements as you settle into the Dragon stance. The waist is still turned a little to the right so that the right arm is extended to the right of the body and the left hand is in front of the left shoulder.

Move 46.

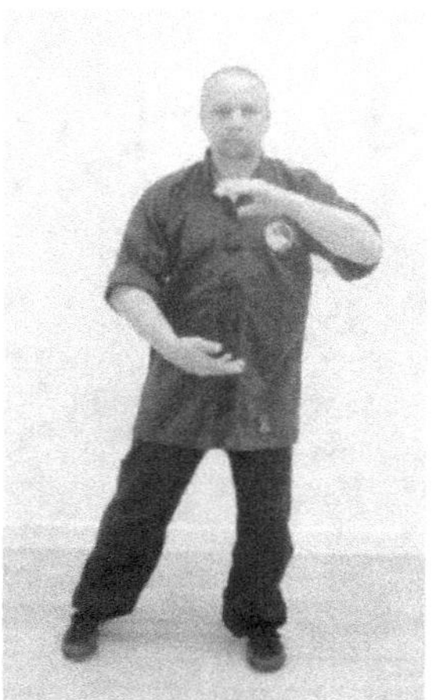

Stance: Left Leopard
Facing: South

<u>Stance movement:</u>

The weight shifts back onto the right foot and then the left foot 'hooks' to point towards the South with the heels of both feet in line with each other. Move the weight onto the left leg and correct the right foot to come into Leopard stance.

<u>Posture movement:</u>

The right hand circles out to the right and then down before continuing its circle to come in front of the body at waist height (with the palm facing upwards). The left arm 'rolls' with the body so that it finishes with the palm facing downwards. Ensure that both palms are facing each other as if holding a 'ball' in front of the body.

Move 47.

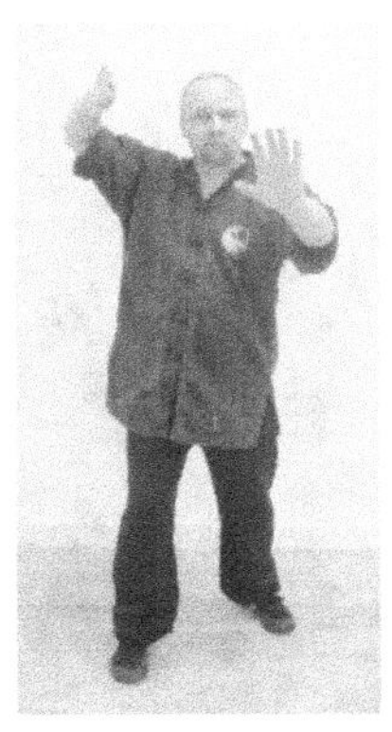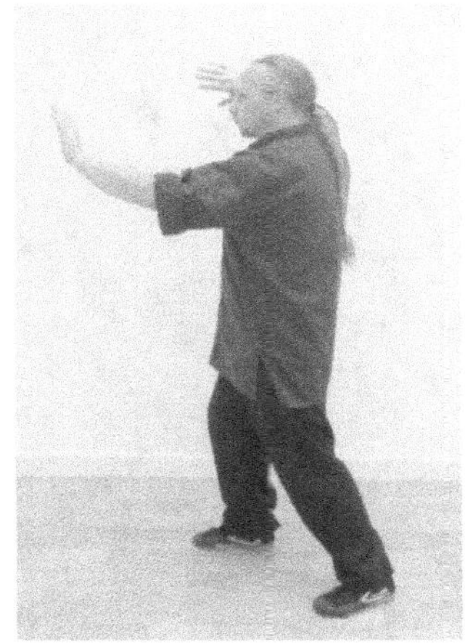

Stance: Right Dragon
Facing: West

<u>Stance movement:</u>

Step the right foot around to point towards the West and then shift the weight onto it before correcting the left foot to finish in Dragon stance.

<u>Posture movement:</u>

Both hands 'roll' with the body so that the right hand draws up and back to finish at head height with the palm facing away from the head and the little finger edge upwards. The left hand circles downwards and then forwards and back up to shoulder height extended to the front with the palm facing forwards away from the body. Again, the waist is turned slightly to the right to bring the right hand into the correct position.

Move 48.

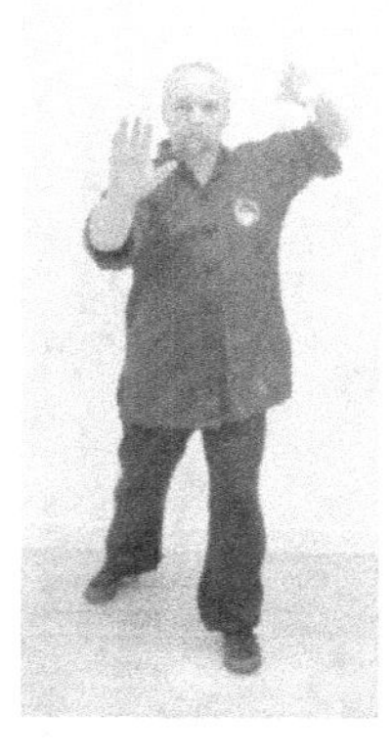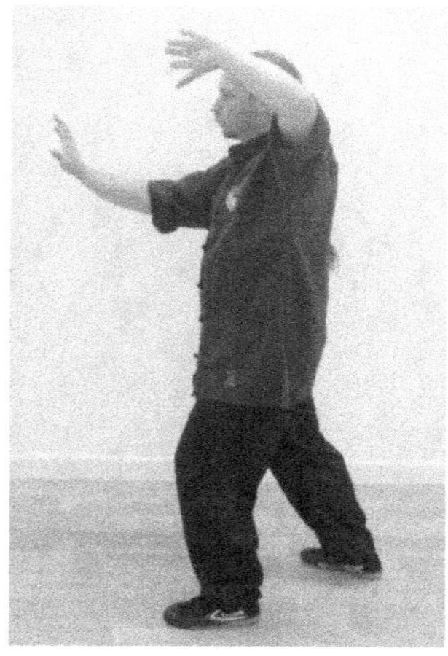

Stance: Left Dragon
Facing: West

<u>Stance movement:</u>

Step the left foot forwards, bringing the weight onto it and correcting the back foot to finish in Dragon stance (so stepping forwards from one Dragon stance to the other).

<u>Posture movement:</u>

The arms roll so as to reverse their positions, so the left hand draws back and up to head height and the right hand rolls down and forwards in a 'palm strike' type movement. The upper body should be turned slightly to the left from the waist.

Move 49.

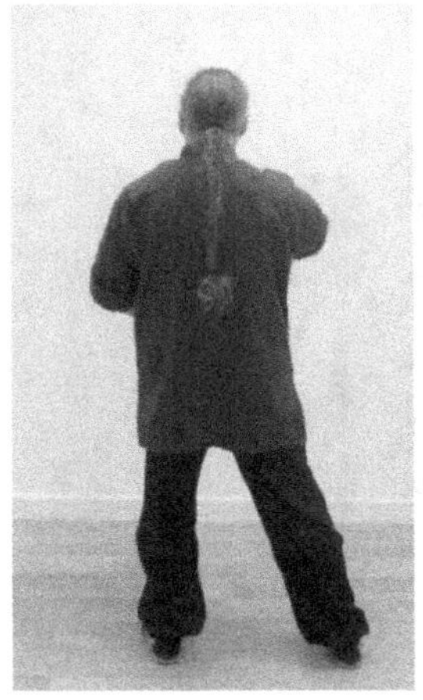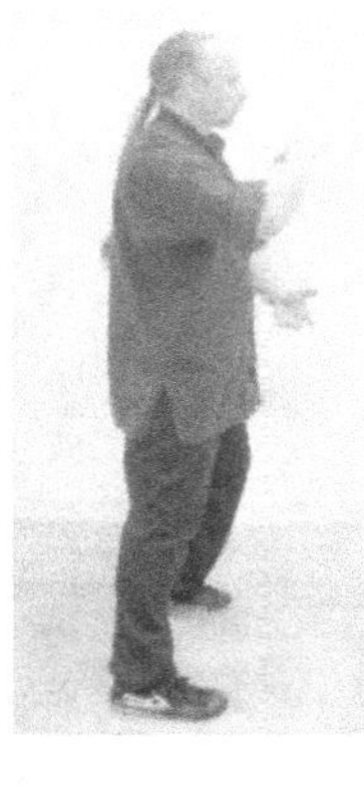

Stance: Left Leopard
Facing: North

<u>Stance movement:</u>

Step the right foot back behind you to bring the heel in line with the left heel and place the foot with the toes facing North. Correct the left foot to also point towards the North (with just a small weight shift to free up the foot) and settle into the Left Leopard stance.

<u>Posture movement:</u>

The right arm rolls downwards and then passes the right hip before continuing the circle (over and inwards) to finish with the palm down in front of the chest. The left arm circles down in front of the body to finish with the palm upwards at Tantien level in front of the body. Note the similarities with movement number Forty-Six.

Move 50.

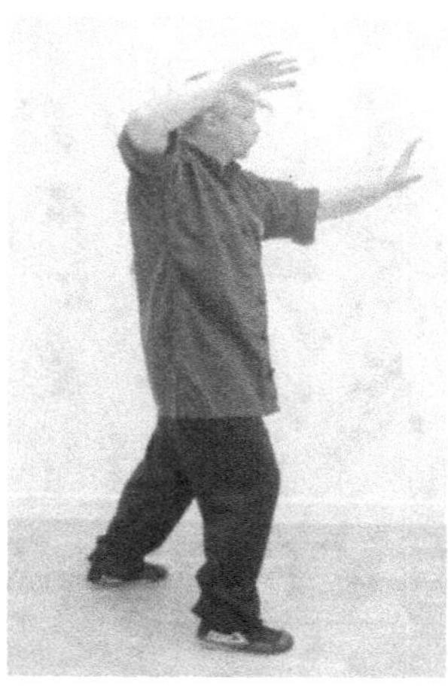

Stance: Right Dragon
Facing: East

<u>Stance movement:</u>

Step the right foot around to your right (pointing the toes towards the East) and then shift the weight onto it and correct the left foot to come into Dragon stance.

<u>Posture movement:</u>

The left hand rolls up and forwards as you come into the Dragon to 'push' forwards with the palm at shoulder height. The right hand rolls up and back to beside the head with the palm facing outwards (little finger edge on top). The waist should be turned a little to the right to bring the right hand into the correct position.

Move 51.

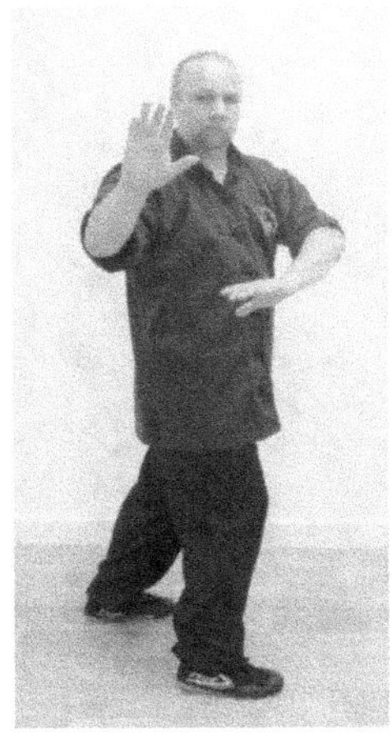 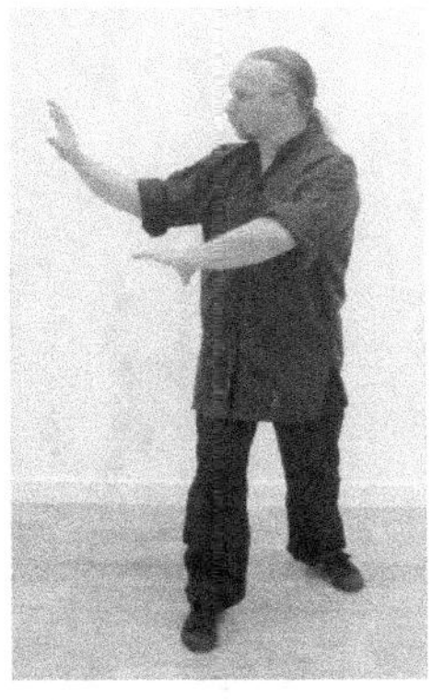

Stance: Right Dragon
Facing: East

<u>Stance movement:</u>

Remain in the same Right Dragon stance throughout this movement.

<u>Posture movement:</u>

Turn the upper body to the right (from the waist so you do not corrupt the stance). The right hand extends outwards with the palm to shoulder height and the left hand comes inwards and across the body to finish palm downwards at around waist height.

Move 52.

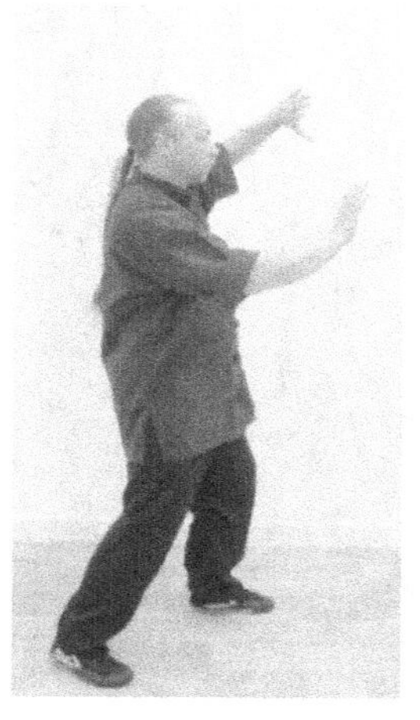 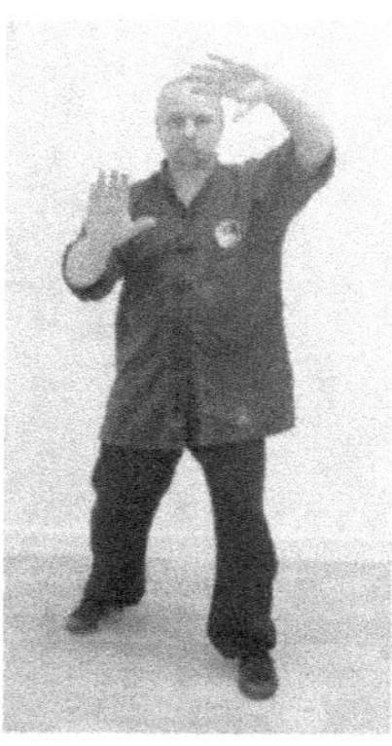

Stance: Left Dragon
Facing: East

<u>Stance movement:</u>

Step through with the left foot and come forwards into Left Dragon stance.

<u>Posture movement:</u>

The left hand draws back and up to finish with the little finger edge upwards and the palm facing forwards at around forehead height – the hand should be extended forward and away from the head. The right hand follows a circle to 'push' forwards with a slight 'underarm' movement to shoulder height extended forwards. Both hands 'roll' through these movements together as you step forwards and straighten the waist.

Move 53.

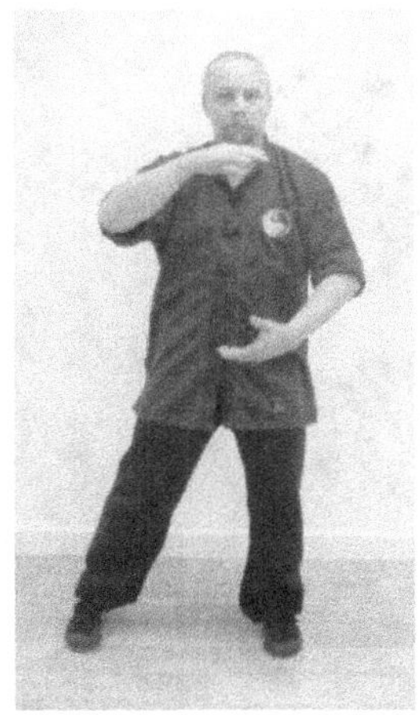

Stance: Left Leopard
Facing: South

<u>Stance movement:</u>

Step the right foot back behind you to place the heel in line with the left heel and the toes pointing South. Make a small weight shift to correct the left foot and then settle the weight back onto the left foot into the Leopard stance.

<u>Posture movement:</u>

Both arms circle downwards and to the right. The left hand follows the circle to come up in front of the body at waist height with the palm facing upwards and the right hand continues the circle to come up and over to the right side of the body. The right hand then continues the circle further to finish palm downwards in front of the body at chest height, so the hands are holding a 'ball' in front of the body.

<u>Timing:</u>

Both hands and stance should finish simultaneously.

Move 54.

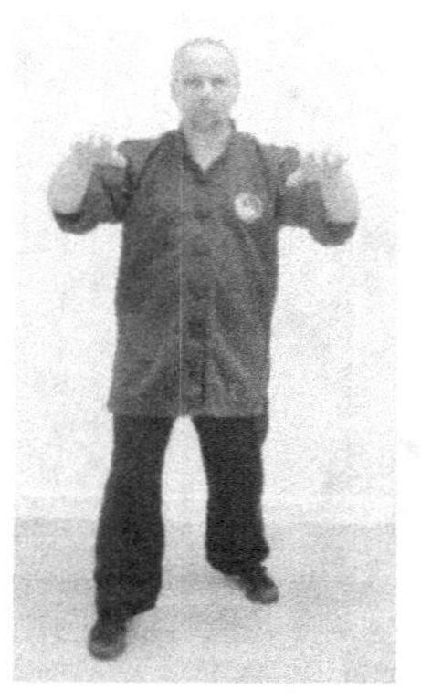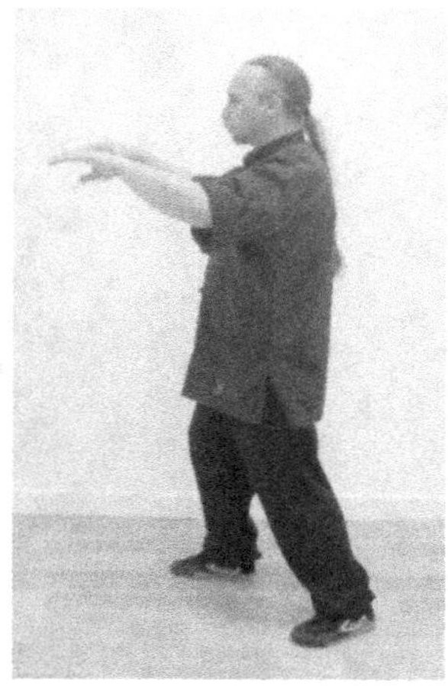

Stance: Right Dragon
Facing: West

<u>Stance movement:</u>

Step the right foot around and to your right before bringing the weight onto it and correcting the back foot to come into Dragon stance facing West.

<u>Posture movement:</u>

Both arms roll down to around waist height in front of the body before 'drifting' up to shoulder height with the palms facing downwards.

Move 55.

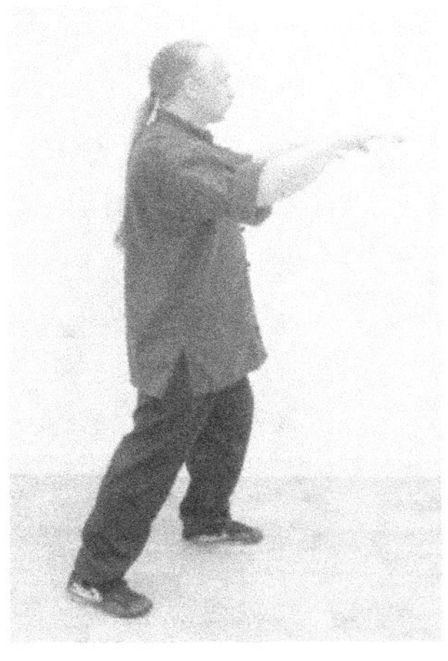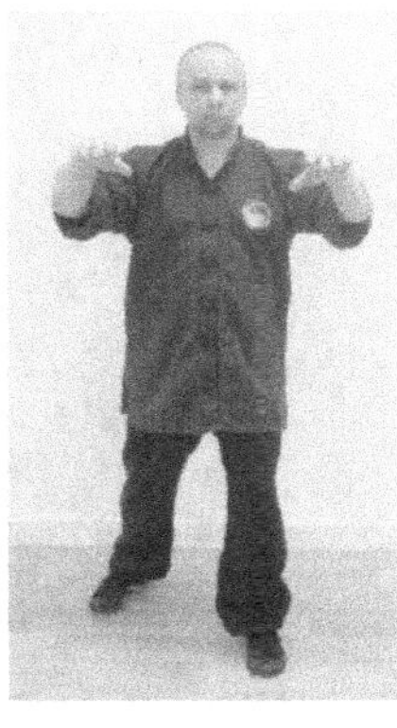

Stance: Left Dragon
Facing: East

<u>Stance movement:</u>

Bring the weight back onto the left leg and then correct the right foot to point the toes towards the South-East. Shift onto the right leg and step the left foot around to the East before moving the weight onto the left foot into Dragon stance.

<u>Posture movement:</u>

The arms drift down in front of the body to waist height and then (as you come into the Left Dragon stance) drift back up to shoulder height to finish with the palms facing downwards once again.

Move 56.

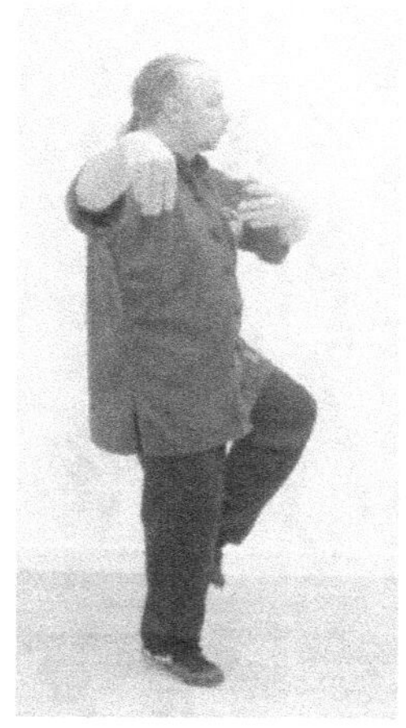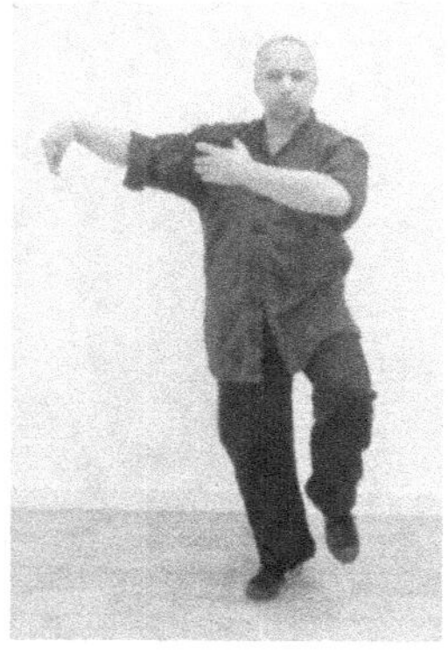

Stance: Left Crane
Facing: East

<u>Stance movement:</u>

Draw your weight back onto the right leg and then lift the left foot up into Crane stance.

<u>Posture movement:</u>

The arms both roll downwards, then turn the waist to the right bringing both arms to the right side of the body. The left arm circles up and inwards to finish with the palm facing in towards the right shoulder. The right arm circles up and outwards to finish by 'rolling' slightly over shoulder height and then down as it comes forwards to finish at shoulder height extended to the right side of the body. The fingers of the right hand 'hang' downwards as it comes up to shoulder height so that the hand is held in the 'Crane's Head' position.

Move 57.

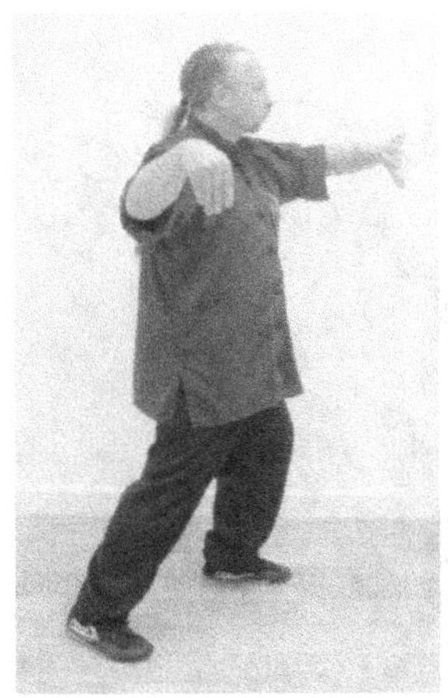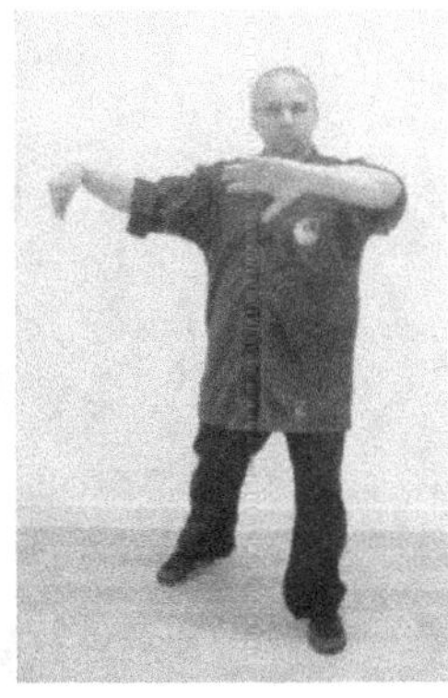

Stance: Left Dragon
Facing: East

<u>Stance movement:</u>

Place the left foot down in front of you and shift the weight forwards onto it into Dragon stance.

<u>Posture movement:</u>

The left hand 'scoops' down and then forwards and up to finish at shoulder height. The right arm rolls in a small 'anti-clockwise' circle at shoulder height. The waist is still turned to the right so that the right arm is extended to the side and the left hand is across the chest.

Move 58.

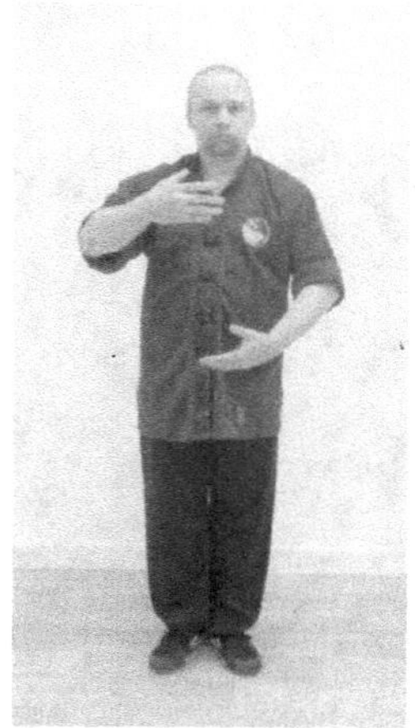

Stance: Eagle
Facing: South

<u>Stance movement:</u>

Draw the weight back onto the right foot enough to be able to correct the left foot to point towards the South-East. Move back onto the left foot and step the right foot in so that you come into an Eagle stance facing South.

<u>Posture movement:</u>

The right arm circles back and down before coming up in front of the body with the palm facing inwards to chest height. The left hand rolls down and in to in front of the body at waist height with the palm facing upwards. This position is often referred to as 'holding the baby'!

Move 59.

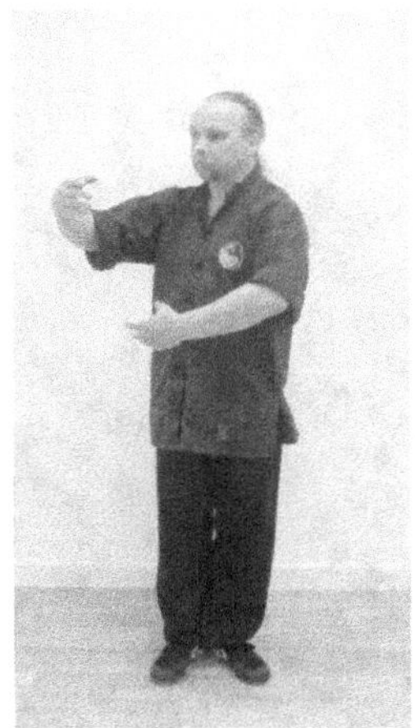

Stance: Eagle
Facing: South

Stance movement:

Remain in the Eagle stance during this movement.

Posture movement:

Turn the upper body (from the waist) to your right (to around a forty-five degree angle). Both hands move slightly further away from the body and the left hand turns to bring the palm more towards the body. (This movement is usually referred to as 'rocking the baby'.)

Move 60.

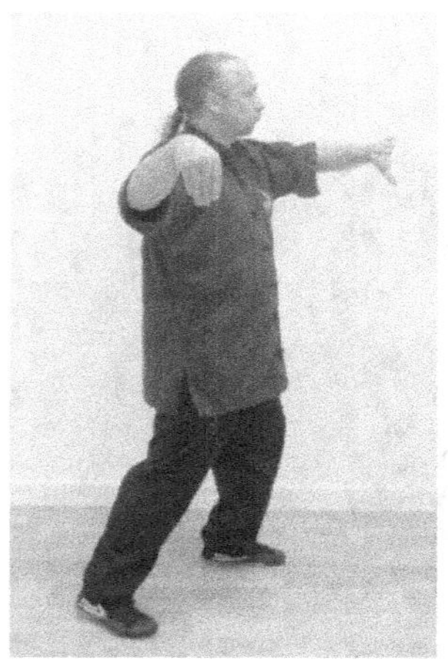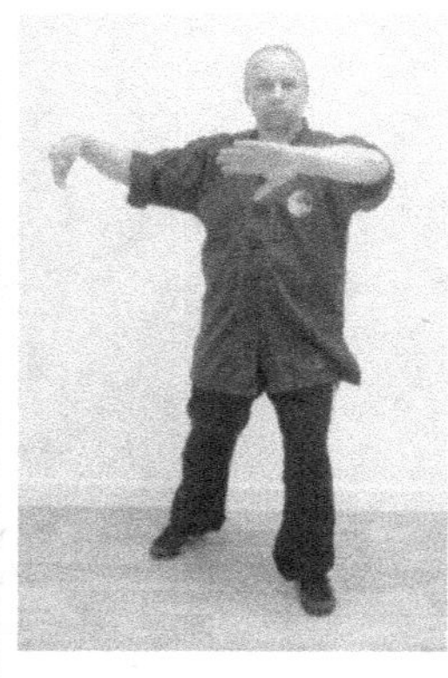

Stance: Left Dragon
Facing: East

<u>Stance movement:</u>

Step the left foot around to your left and turn ninety degrees to the left into Dragon stance.

<u>Posture movement:</u>

The left hand 'scoops' up and outwards to shoulder height extended forwards in front of the body. The right arm draws a small 'anti-clockwise' circle at shoulder height to finish once again in a 'Crane's Head' position extended out to the right (with the waist turned to the right slightly).

Afterword:
A comment from the author.

The majority of you, reading this book, will probably have been training in Lee Family Style Tai Chi for a number of years now and I hope that this volume will be helpful for you as you continue to train these wonderful and truly holistic Arts. The longer you train, the more you realise that there is still left to learn – that stills holds true for me after all the years that I have put into these Arts and that is where much of the pleasure of the continued training comes from.

I have gained enormous benefits from my studies of Lee Family Tai Chi and I have thoroughly enjoyed my time training with some amazing people.

Keep practicing and I look forward to sharing more of my personal Tai Chi journey with you all.

Conrad Robinson, 2021

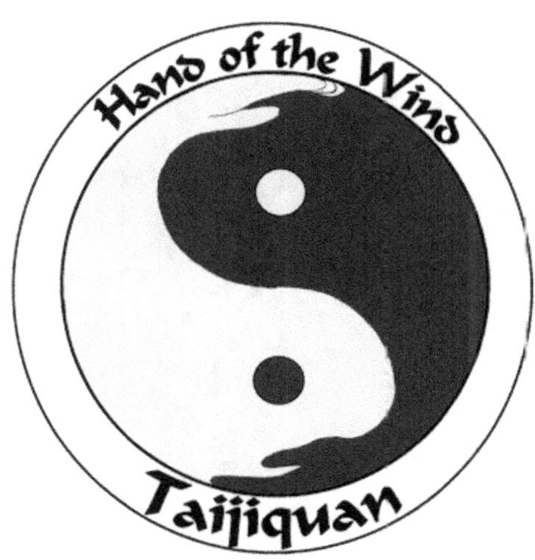

Notes:

Notes:

Notes